SOUNDS OF *TOHI*

SOUNDS OF *TOHI*
VᎧ OᏃZET

Cherokee Health and Well-Being
in Southern Appalachia

DhᏌSGᎩ OᏃZᎧGᏒ VᎧ DSᎷᏏ
GWᎩ OᏊᎧᏗ VᎥᎦT

LISA J. LEFLER AND THOMAS N. BELT (CHEROKEE)

FOREWORD BY PAMELA DUNCAN

FOREWORD BY T. J. HOLLAND
(EASTERN BAND OF CHEROKEE INDIANS)

AFTERWORD BY TOM HATLEY

THE UNIVERSITY OF ALABAMA PRESS   TUSCALOOSA

The University of Alabama Press
Tuscaloosa, Alabama 35487-0380
uapress.ua.edu

Typeface: Minion Pro

Cover image: T. J. Holland, *The Phrenology of Judaculla*, oil on
canvas, 2011; courtesy of Caroline P. Holland
Cover design: Michele Myatt Quinn

Cataloging-in-Publication data is available from the Library of Congress.
ISBN: 978-0-8173-2119-2
E-ISBN: 978-0-8173-9415-8

To my sisters, Janice L. Reed and Diane Lefler, through whom I can see the faith and strength of our mother running like the Tuckasegee River after a hard summer storm, and to all women of Appalachia who give us hope and direction. Thank you.

LISA J. LEFLER

To my mother and father, Mattie and Cooweescowee Belt, to continue the world through their eyes.

THOMAS N. BELT

A special dedication to T. J. Holland (1976–2020), whose words and artistic creativity are reflected in this volume. He lived his life to preserve the culture of his people and to serve all. His generosity of knowledge and self will be remembered.

THOMAS N. BELT AND LISA J. LEFLER

CONTENTS

Foreword
Pamela Duncan ix

Foreword
T. J. Holland xi

Preface
Lisa J. Lefler xiii

Introduction 1

Chapter One
Tohi (ᏫᏙᎯ) 10

Chapter Two
Making a Connection between Indigenous Women, History, and
Healing the Community: A Brief Introduction to Matrilineality 16

Chapter Three
When the Land Is Sick, We Are Sick: Metaphysics
of Indigenous Epistemologies 29

Chapter Four
The Land Keeps Our History and Identity: Cherokee
and Appalachian Cosmography 39

Chapter Five
Indigenizing Counseling 50

Chapter Six
We Are *of* This Place: Integrating Traditional Science and Health 63

Chapter Seven
Decolonizing and Indigenizing Our Minds for Better Health: *Tohi* 71

Afterword: Listening to the Sounds of *Tohi*
Tom Hatley 82

Acknowledgments 87

Further Reading 89

References 91

Index 97

FOREWORD

I first met Lisa Lefler in 2003 when I visited City Lights Bookstore in Sylva, North Carolina, to do a reading from my second novel, *Plant Life*. Right away I felt a kinship not only because she was so friendly and welcoming, but also because she was so proud of our shared mountain heritage and culture. We swapped stories and compared our experiences as Appalachians in a world that all too often misunderstood or belittled our people, our talk, our way of life. She took me to meet her mama, Jean Lefler, the epitome of a mountain woman: someone wise, strong, and loving; a healer; a spiritual human who deeply valued our connection to the land and mourned the damage caused by human greed and corruption. A few years later, Lisa introduced me to her friend Tom Belt, a Cherokee elder and first-language speaker and teacher. Tom is a funny guy, a great storyteller, but behind that lightheartedness, he shares with Lisa and Jean the same abiding love and concern for the land and the culture of these mountains. Most of my adult life had been lived away from the mountains, but Lisa, Jean, and Tom reminded me of who I was, where I came from, where I belonged. And when I moved to Cullowhee in 2008 to teach at Western Carolina University, I knew I was finally home, back in the mountains where I was born, back with people who shared a love for our place, our history, and our culture.

In a 1985 *New York Times* essay, "Where I Ought to Be: A Writer's Sense of Place," author Louise Erdrich states: "Once we no longer live beneath our mother's heart, it is the earth with which we form the same dependent relationship, relying completely on its cycles and elements, helpless without its protective embrace." The truth of that statement—for all of us, not just Cherokees and Appalachians—is explored and explained in this book through the lens of *tohi*, or Cherokee health and well-being. *Tohi* encompasses all aspects of good health—physical, mental, emotional, and spiritual—and emphasizes the interconnectedness of the land and its people as necessary for the good health of both. Lisa, a medical anthropologist, has spent her professional life immersed in the study of the culture, health, and medicine of Native populations and believes strongly in the value of practical applications of ancient ways of knowing and healing. As an elder and a native speaker, Tom is a walking encyclopedia of the concepts and origins of Cherokee medicine that are embedded in the language and culture of the Kituwah (DhⱯSGⱯ) people. Now more than ever we need their voices, their experience, their wisdom. Poet Maurice Manning (2006) says, "What troubles humans most is their desire to remove themselves from Nature." So much of the sickness of people and the environment can be attributed to this distance between us and the natural world. By sharing their stories and their knowledge, Lisa and Tom offer remedies for that distance, that sickness.

This book is a continuation of a conversation begun many years ago in the home of Jean Lefler, a conversation between Appalachians and Cherokees; between friends, healers, and scholars. I can think of no one better suited to write a book about the healing power of connection to place, language, and culture than Lisa and Tom. And while Jean is no longer with us in this world, I believe she is the guiding spirit of this book, a spirit that invites you to sit on the porch with her to listen and to learn from these mountain voices.

PAMELA DUNCAN
SYLVA, NORTH CAROLINA

FOREWORD

I've had the pleasure of knowing and working with Tom and Lisa for sixteen years. In that time there has been many a conference, presentation, or tour that involved one or the both of them. Since we're all averse to flying, we've logged countless hours on the road and countless words in conversation. I do more listening than talking, considering I can't learn anything if my mouth is open. In addition to solving the world's problems, we discussed the concepts in this volume, exploring them for hours on end. Whether we were talking about history, culture, or personal experiences, every topic we discussed seemed to relate to the importance of place.

There are countless Cherokee stories, and almost every one occurs in a specific place. These stories taken together form a cosmography that when understood, defines Cherokee culture. They tell us not only who we are, but how we are to relate to our surroundings, and how we are to treat one another. Our stories teach us that we are not rugged individualists; we are part of a community, connected to the land and one another.

For Native and mountain people alike, a sense of community is often taken for granted. We grow up with grandparents, aunts, and uncles around us living no more than a short drive away. We go to school with our cousins. Family friends extend over generations. On some level, no matter specific cultural backgrounds, the mountains provide and shape a worldview. These mountains are not a place to be *from*, but a place to be *of*.

Tom has talked about growing up in Oklahoma, and speaking in the Cherokee language using the terms "uphill" (ᏍᏑᎤᎦᏬ) and "downhill" (ᏛᎤᏬᏍᏬ) even though the places being referenced are generally flat. The Cherokee language's formation in the mountains dictates the spatial orientation, no matter where it is spoken.

At this point in history, the Cherokee people have shared these homelands with people of European and African descent for over four hundred years. Generations of Appalachian white people and African Americans have lived and learned in the same mountains, and both have experienced the effects of stereotyping by a dominant culture. As mountain people, we know that these mountains, and the places in them, can provide the answers to many of the problems that we deal with in today's world.

This book has been written by two people who are *of* a place. They understand their connection to the world through their place in it. I ask you, the reader, not to interpret this volume, but to just listen. The lessons that Lisa and Tom are teaching can apply to any people who are of a place.

T. J. HOLLAND
SNOWBIRD COMMUNITY, GRAHAM COUNTY, NORTH CAROLINA

PREFACE

Little has been written about Appalachian and Cherokee histories as interconnected in a positive, symbiotic way. I hope that this book can add to an understanding of how people from these different yet connected histories and heritages have learned from each other, listened to each other, and respected their similarities and differences. Both are cultures steeped in negative stereotypes ensconced in the national consciousness, which still plague them and have serious social and environmental consequences. These stereotypes can be easily traced back to three groups just before and after the turn of the twentieth century: local-color writers, home missions, and educators who wanted to raise critical funds from wealthy businessmen up north to continue their work. Herb Smith's great film *Strangers and Kin: A History of the Hillbilly Image* (1984) is a wonderful reference that reflects each group's contributions to these damning and irrepressible images.

Events coincided with these groups' arrival to create a perfect storm that solidified these notions about who Appalachian people were. Notions such as dialect equating to ignorance, incestuous and clannish families, violent mountain folks, and a host of other negative images were repeated and reiterated in media, literature, and even early silent film (McCarroll 2018). Many of the ideas about mountain people as peculiar or strange flourished from the seeds of a mixed loyalty during the Civil War, politicians who rationalized the extreme poverty that affected the Appalachian region after the war, the yellow journalism that covered the news of the time, and the use of all of these stereotypes by news outlets, writers, missionaries, and government officials, all of whom had a vested interest in their creation and perpetuation.

More importantly, however, the longitudinal impact of these stereotypes has created a foundation of justification and rationale for the discriminatory treatment of mountain people for generations. This is clearly evident in major governmental removal events such as those mandated for the projects of the Tennessee Valley Authority, the establishment of various parks such as the Shenandoah and Great Smoky Mountains, and the construction of the Blue Ridge Parkway (Perdue and Martin-Perdue 1979–80). These examples pale in comparison of course to the government-mandated Removal of Native peoples in 1838.

Thankfully, however, there are those within these populations who work diligently to contradict those images and concentrate their energies on fostering resiliency and a more positive future, such as the documentarians of Appalshop and the many scholars who produce hard research and present each year at the Appalachian Studies Association conference, a good number of whom are products of Appalachia themselves. A wonderful recent edited volume, *Appalachian Reckoning* (Harkins and McCarroll 2019), reflects the diversity, energy, and resiliency of the people of Appalachia, challenging the monolithic, victim-blaming, more highly touted volume of J. D. Vance's, *Hillbilly Elegy* (2016). The podcast *The Bitter Southerner* hosted a great discussion of how the 2019 volume illuminates *Hillbilly Elegy*'s negative impact on the people of Appalachia (see Reece 2020).

To counter the negative stereotypes and monolithic presentations that have left only shallow and diminished ideas of Appalachia, we would like to share the interactions and work of two people whose roots run deep in these mountains: Tom Belt, a Cherokee elder and first-language speaker, and myself, a woman who grew up in and out of the mountains but was always connected there through the words and actions of my mother. We are speaking not for the people of Appalachia, but only for ourselves, and for the way that our connectedness to place by our ancestors has forged our identity as mountain people. In this volume, Tom's stories, linguistic expertise, and cultural understanding are included from recorded interviews and my field notes along with varied conversations. His comments are in quotation marks as examples of why language preservation is an urgent priority for Native communities.

The aim of this book is to draw from the experiences and culture of this region so as to reflect how connected we all are to one another and to the world around us. We can heal by being connected to place, language, and culture. By honoring our families, land, and heritage we gain a sense of continuity over generations that root and solidify who we are. We learn from our ancestors and our neighbors how to respect the land and others, strengthening ourselves in the process. This is a critical time in our world's history, when we are witness to climate change and rapid and widespread destruction of our natural resources. We find ourselves being pulled apart from our humanity and sense of connectedness by a politics of hatred and the demonization of those who are different. There are forces in our world that seek to divide us, and this loss of connection fuels that division.

My family's roots are deeply embedded in Southern Appalachia, and my earliest memories are about living in a small, four-room cabin with no in-door plumbing and a pipe positioned through the kitchen wall that allowed a constant flow of fresh, clean spring water into the sink. I remember sneaking past the rock canning house up the hill to the outhouse, keeping an eye out for the copperheads sidled up to the walls for warmth. During the warm months I learned to hold going to the bathroom at night so I wouldn't have to venture out in the dark and navigate the spiders and snakes. I remember my mom taking us up the mountain to learn about what trees and plants grew near and how to identify them when their leaves were off, and what they could provide us when someone was sick, hurt, or hungry. I played with the crawdads and salamanders in the creek by the house as if they were close friends who would meet me after school. I was always amazed by the multitude of mosses and ferns, which provided my play space with bedding and carpeting for a cozy place to hide out. The vast array of quartz, granite, mica, and other rocks provided endless hours of building and organizing and, when washed, shined a multitude of colors.

My days were full of running and walking the mountainsides and hollers, imagining being a cowboy on a Morgan horse or a hunter tracking a panther (we called them painters). Even in a household where my father battled alcoholism and the trauma of an abandoned childhood and my mother worked for little to nothing in a sewing plant and had childhood traumas and abandonment of her own, I learned that emotional and psychological refuge could be found in those beautiful, mysterious, and wondrous mountains. Being there, in those mountains, was healing. Being there made us whole.

Born during the Depression, my mother was the oldest of five children. Her family was an anomaly in that her mother and father divorced. Soon after the divorce, she inherited the responsibilities of an adult when her mother turned the children out to fend for themselves though my mother herself was not yet a teenager. With no money and no home, Mom had to take care of herself and her siblings. She learned early on that the mountains could take care of you but you had to be conscious of what they had to teach. She learned how to hunt and gather for food and medicine. She found value in the serenity of listening to the water in rivers and streams, and praying on the highest ridges, closest to God for peace and guidance. She listened to elders explain not to be afraid but learn from the earth and the creatures that lived here, and recognize that we all have a purpose.

As an adult, thanks to this difficult experience, she was always known for her knowledge of the region and her ability to grow anything. She was also known for her sense of peace and spirituality, qualities I always attributed to her continual connection with place. Not just any place but specifically the mountains of western North Carolina.

It wasn't until I was about seven or eight years old that the reality of what she knew, particularly about plants, became crystal clear. My dad had been down east on a job and had gotten a systemic blood infection that manifested in oozing sores on his legs that wouldn't heal. As soon as he got home, Mom took him to see Doc Mitchell over in Bryson City. Doc Mitchell was a living legend in this area and had doctored most everyone in three counties. He was in charge of the local hospital and was known as a man who took his profession seriously.

When the doctor examined Dad, he told us that he had diabetes and that this infection would cause my father to lose his legs. This was the first time I ever saw my father cry. My mother, seeing the toll it was taking on my father, told Doc Mitchell that she wanted to take Dad home and see whether she could help before they agreed to amputations. "I'll bring him back in two days if I can't help him," she said. So we loaded Dad back in the car and took him home, and Mom gave us a list of what she needed. We took off up the mountain and brought back slippery elm and the combination of other botanicals she had instructed us to collect. She combined the barks, roots, and plants and boiled them into poultices that she placed on his legs night and day for the next forty-eight hours. Her work made it possible for him to keep his legs for another thirty years. My siblings and I remember many other instances where she was able to intervene by both her knowledge and her faith.

My father was characterized by his wanderlust; he was a rolling stone constantly searching for something else. His alcoholism made it difficult to hold down a steady job, so he often traveled throughout the South and across the state in search of work, identity, and a drink. Often he would insist that we come with him and because Mom believed her duty was to keep the family together and follow her husband, she would pack us up and off we would go. Usually we would end up in a trailer park or insecure housing, or occasionally the car. We would be there until he lost his job or until Mom could scrape enough money together to get back home.

As we approached the mountains, whether it was coming toward Black Mountain from the east or coming up Saluda from the south, my eyes would begin to water and my heart felt as though it was going to burst in my chest at sight of the first mountain peak. I was elated that we were home. I knew that here, things were going to be okay. People here talked like me. I would not be made fun of for the way I spoke, or thought of as white trash because our clothes were all handmade. I didn't feel like a fish out of water. I was home. The terrain was familiar. I didn't feel exposed. The mountains were like arms that held me close and safe.

Being taken from a place of familiarity repeatedly shook me to my core. It meant being taken from a place where I knew my family for generations had lived, where those roots to place made me more connected. Even though I learned a lot from moving around, changing schools, and making friends here and there, I knew that my identity, my stability, came from being back in those mountains of my family. Each time, leaving was incredibly painful and traumatic. There was a sadness that I felt could never be overcome, at least not until our return. I felt fragmented and spiritually rootless. Even though we were regular churchgoers, my church, my place for thinking about and speaking to God, was outside. That's where God was. God was in the sky, the wind, the water, the rocks, the trees, and even the ground cover. In the mountains God was all around me. I think this was what made me feel comfortable and connected in my work with Native peoples. This is why the conversations in those years I spent visiting with folks from Cherokee and other tribes made sense in ways more often than did the worldview of non-Natives. Both Cherokee and those non-Natives who settled in these mountains are all Appalachian—that is, people of the mountains. This is where we intersect. This is our common ground.

After my father passed away, my mom moved in with me. It would not be uncommon for me to come home and find Mom visiting with ladies she had worked with in the sewing plant. Some were Cherokee, and they often would be talking about plants, changing weather, and the way things were growing up. A few years before she passed, an old friend, Cherokee elder Tom Belt, would often come by for a visit and they would talk about all things mountain. She never tired of talking about how she grew up, asking Tom about how he grew up in Oklahoma, and sharing stories of both hardships and fun. Mom would share what was most meaningful about being a mountain woman, and Tom about being Cherokee. Humor was always a large part of it.

Their visits were so engaging that as we knew Mom was nearing the end of her life, we felt it important that these dialogues continue and reflect the understanding that connected this Appalachian woman and Cherokee elder. The talks about what guided them, preserved them, helped them be resilient—that, and acknowledging the sacred—needed to continue and be shared with more who were like-minded and like-spirited.

Through these exchanges I became more and more aware of the language and teachings of the Cherokee, or Kituwah, people. Tom explained how concepts of medicine, health, healing, doctoring, and origins of medicine in the Cherokee way were all part of interconnected systems of how to live, how to think, and how to be a human being within the cultural epistemologies of Kituwah people. Significantly, these concepts, preserved for millennia in the language of Kituwahs, have practical applications for us today as is exemplified in the coming chapter on counseling. It is a language of people who identify themselves literally as "people of the earth, of the dirt that belongs to the Creator." The language connects them with place, with the mountains of western North Carolina, with the earth, and it will provide others who settled here with a connectedness as well.

Tom says he and my mother both had seats on the porch; he referred to the mountains as the porch from which they both sat and viewed the world. He said he could talk with her as though he had known her his whole life. There was a familiarity about her and the way they communicated with each other. They were both grounded in what the mountains taught them. There was healing in that way of thinking and talking, and that is the gift of being part of the mountains. He said, "People here are given a label, a wrapper that makes you think of them in only one way but doesn't reflect what is inside. Inside, being a part of the mountains makes you whole. Understanding that connectedness to such a diverse and beautiful place also has a responsibility with it. As beautiful as it is, you can easily die out there if you don't pay attention and act in a way that respects what's there. You are of this place, not just from it, and that means you have a relationship with this natural world." Relationships are at the heart of this discussion, as is the need for connection.

In nonindustrialized societies, ideas of tribalism, clannish communities, extended family systems, and group emphasis were, and are, cultural values. Most features of these societies reflect the importance of recognizing others to not only survive but thrive and be healthy. For those growing up in a rural area, it didn't take a rocket scientist to understand how much we needed one another to live. On subsistence farms, it took many hands and strong backs to do the chores that allowed crops to be grown and harvested, to take care of the animals and process them when time, to properly maintain the home and land, and to share all that had been produced.

After the colonization and industrialization of our society, we began to see a greater emphasis placed on individualism, bolstered by the evangelical Christian belief in a personal relationship with God, which, however strong, diminished community. Industrialization encouraged individualism, a separation from the land, mobility to urban areas, and a shift in thinking from a larger, extended family system to a more nuclear one. We've institutionalized things like taking care of our elders and teaching our children. We have become disassociated with our natural world and relegate that interaction to holidays and vacations. And with that, we lose the healing that comes with these connections to family and place, and even the language that categorizes how we perceive them.

This book is a shared reflection from two people who both value the healing qualities of being rooted, whose identities are grounded to place, not just from our own generation, but from those generations before us who loved these mountains and considered them part of their soul, and who, when they passed, became part of these mountains, buried deep in their soil. There is a wholeness in that, a healing that comes full circle and allows us to be saturated in the warmth and comfort of some of the oldest geological features in the world.

Agrarian philosopher and poet Wendell Berry (2002) wrote, "To think better, to think like the best humans, we are probably going to have to learn again to judge a person's intelligence, not by the ability to recite facts, but by the good order or harmoniousness of his or her surroundings" (192–93). He was referring to one's relationship with the land, and an understanding of the importance of being good stewards. He too sees one's relationship with the land and environment as critical to good health, both mental and physical.

I have known many who, in their adolescence and young adulthood, fought to escape the mountains and longed for the busy, active life of urban living. They wanted to separate themselves from what the popular culture's images of Appalachia said they were, what they didn't have the words or energy to refute. But most of those very people in their later years felt homesick for the mountains of their childhood. They didn't feel fully whole, displaced by a lifestyle disconnected from nature and the community it reflected. So in "coming home" they were able to regain parts of themselves that reminded them of that important relationship to something larger than themselves, something dynamic, something beautiful. They could relate to an identity and heritage that was their own and reflected qualities of tenaciousness and the victory of survival. For many, a life of hardship became memories of how families and communities came together in bad and good times. We learned the lessons of sharing, working hard, and playing hard. We learned to listen, to watch, and to be grateful for the never-ending beauty and mysteries of the mountains.

I think of my old family friends Mary Jane Queen and her older sister, Ella, mountain women who never met a stranger. They treated everyone with joy and respect, never had a harsh word for anyone, and loved their home place of Caney Fork, which lies above the Cherokee sacred carved rock, Judaculla, the largest petroglyph in the eastern United States. Even in their late eighties, they would successfully race me up the mountain to collect buck berries, and gleefully chide me for being unable to keep up. Mary Jane and Ella's family were incredible musicians who entertained on the back porch of their home on a mountaintop and could play all night and never repeat a mountain ballad. Mary Jane had notebooks full of ballads and songs that had been handed down in their family over hundreds of years. They both worked hard and played hard and had a love for wildflowers, waterfalls, and family. They were the epitome of mountain women. They were whole, happy, and healthy. To think of them apart from the mountains was impossible for anyone who knew them.

One day I took Tom to visit Mary Jane, and he saw that she, too, was familiar in the way my mom was. They got to talking about plants and animals, and they got around to talking about rattlesnakes. Tom told her that Cherokees held them in great respect; they had the power of life and death, and it was traditional to speak to them. He asked her what she would do if she saw one. Her response was simply, "I'm not sure what I would say to one. But I'm sure it would be something short."

People like Tom's parents and grandparents, my mom, Mary Jane, and Ella are all great examples of people of the mountains. Tom's parents and grandparents didn't grow up in North Carolina, but were victims of Removal in 1838. His ancestors were removed from Shooting Creek in Macon County, North Carolina, and walked the Trail of Tears to Oklahoma. I had the unexpected, very powerful experience of going with Tom to a section of the original Trail of Removal along the Unicoi Turnpike to Fort Armistead near Tellico Plains, Tennessee. Walking that short length of the trail that led his family out of their paradise, their homeland, to the unknown, and that left a legacy of trauma and displacement that was passed on, was unexpectedly formidable for him. It was as though you could feel a pervasive sadness move through that core kinesthetic part of me in a way that overwhelmed my brain. I can't remotely imagine how much more Tom felt the lasting spirit of dread and suffering from the hundreds that walked that very path, many of whom were his family.

Tom spoke of how his parents and grandparents would talk about the place of Kituwah back in North Carolina as though they had lived there. He said, "I heard stories from my grandmother saying there were mountains to the south and east of the ancient town. There is a river that runs along the land. There are seven mountaintops that surround the valley, and the sun makes its journey up the long ridgeline during the summer and then comes back down it in the winter. She said there were four springs that come off four of the mountains into the river. She spoke of it as though she had seen it herself, but she hadn't. These were oral histories, passed down for 150 years. We didn't know exactly where it was. We didn't even know if it was in Tennessee or Georgia or North Carolina, it was just called back home, or where we all came from."

Tom came to Cherokee when he was about twenty-four years old to play the traditional Cherokee game of stickball. He didn't see much, just the grounds where the games were played and the main street of Cherokee. He didn't return until he was in his early forties. He had met Roseanna, an Eastern Band Cherokee woman that he eventually married, and came back to live with her in North Carolina in the 1990s. He said during the time he spent here thirty years earlier, people didn't speak of Kituwah. Most of the people he met then were young people. When he came back he thought about that place his grandmother had spoken of and asked some of the older men about the ancient town. He said,

I saw some old men sitting in front of the Qualla Market. I stopped and asked them about a valley farm down the road. I didn't know who they were, but they were speaking in Cherokee. I asked them in the language if they knew where this place was. I told them who I was, and they responded to my speaking in Cherokee. I asked them about a long valley that I had driven by that was filled with cornfields. One of them said, yes, they call it Governor's Island, but the old people called it Kituwah. It was an old town. That was it! I'd never heard of any other town named Kituwah, and I knew there was only one. This had to be it! I got back in my car and immediately drove back to the pull-off next to the fields. This was a private farm. The Cherokees had lost ownership at Removal. So I looked at the lay of the land and saw the mound, the rise in the earth with corn growing on it, but I knew what it was. The mountains and river were just as my grandmother had told me. This was it. It came alive. I was stunned. I lived just down the road! This was like coming across an old family heirloom. This was that place that had been spoken of for generations in my family. This place of stories became a reality. This is the ground of my ancestors. It was old and it was new to me all at the same time. At that moment I knew I didn't have to look anymore for those things we ask about that make us understand who we are. I knew that this was a living place that would bring peace and comfort and wholeness. There is a difference between a memory and a historical fact. This discovery of place made me really feel Kituwah. I felt I had come home. I took a deep breath and released it with new life.

They had passed on the sacredness and particulars of that place so clearly that when Tom drove by it he stopped and knew immediately that it was Kituwah. There were no signs or identification at that time, before the Tribe's repossession of the mother town in the late 1990s. He said he could feel it and he knew it as though he had visited it every day just by their description. They had kept the knowledge and emotional awareness of the mountains within them even though they had never been back home. He too had a physical response in coming back to the North Carolina mountains, the first of his family since 1838. He felt whole. He had finally come home. He had come home for his parents and grandparents. That is the healing power of place.

LISA J. LEFLER
DILLSBORO, NORTH CAROLINA

SOUNDS OF *TOHI*

INTRODUCTION

When despair for the world grows in me
and I wake in the night at the least sound
in fear of what my life and my children's lives may be,
I go and lie down where the wood drake
rests in his beauty on the water, and the great heron feeds.
I come into the peace of wild things
who do not tax their lives with forethought
of grief. I come into the presence of still water.
And I feel above me the day-blind stars
waiting with their light. For a time
I rest in the grace of the world, and am free.

"THE PEACE OF WILD THINGS," WENDELL BERRY

"The Peace of Wild Things" by the poet and writer Wendell Berry expresses the heart of many who have lived in the oldest mountains in the world, of those who have fished in, sat beside, and gazed at the oldest rivers and streams in the world. Although I do not speak for all Appalachian people, nor Tom for all Native or even Cherokee people, we do share an identity and connection to these mountains and rivers that touch our very soul. In this book we seek where the intersection of our cultures and histories lay and how we see in it the forces that allow resiliency and success to live our lives hopefully with joy, service, and a purpose with others. *They bring us tohi.*

In Charles King's wonderful book *Gods of the Upper Air* (2019), he describes the early students of anthropology at the turn of the twentieth century under the tutelage of Franz Boas, the father of American anthropology. King writes,

They were scientists and thinkers in love with the challenge of understanding other human beings. The deepest science of humanity, they believed, was not one that taught us what was rooted and unchangeable about human nature. Rather, it was the one that revealed the wide variation in human societies—the immense and diverse vocabulary of propriety, custom, morals, and rectitude. Our most cherished traditions, they insisted, are only a tiny fraction of the many ways humans have devised for solving basic problems, from how to order society to how to mark the passage from childhood to adulthood. Just as the cure for a fatal disease might lie in an undiscovered plant in some remote jungle, so too the solution to social problems might be found in how other people in other places have worked out humanity's common challenges. And there is an urgency in this work: as countries change and the world becomes more connected, the catalog of human solutions necessarily gets thinner and thinner. (11)

I would include that with the lack of understanding and value we have placed on those Indigenous, colonized communities, and the lack of respect and understanding that leads to viewing all Appalachian people as backward hillbillies, we have ignored many things that might help us move closer to that goal of knowing how to value and respect all people, all living things, and how to take seriously our relationships with them, improving our own lots in this life.

On a recent webinar sponsored by the National Institute on Alcohol Abuse and Alcoholism (2020), research with the Yup'ik of Alaska was highlighted as a prevention program targeting Native youth. This was a tribal model that engaged the whole community and put culture at the center of the program. One Alaska Native researcher involved in the project started her statements by encouraging us to "bring empathy to our scientific endeavors" and to emphasize the "need for science to be spiritually centered." This was a clear example of an Indigenous community taking the serious problems of substance abuse and suicide head on with the intent to make culture the core of treatment and prevention. It has taken more than five hundred years of colonial occupation for us to get to a point where we in the academy, in particular, listen to and take Indigenous language and culture seriously, understanding that these can offer the strengths for their people to conquer these social pathologies.

Language, culture, and ceremony provide the tools that allow people to believe in themselves, that allow people to become whole and attain real health or *tohi*. For those whose culture and language or dialect come out of the Appalachian Mountains, they too have hundreds of years of negative imagery and discrimination to overcome if they are to make *wanting* to be a positive and resilient people a reality. It is hard to make good decisions about yourself when you think you are, to any degree, less than.

This book is the result of many years of discussion, field notes, events, and networking with others who are interested in traditional knowledge and whose identity is connected to the land. The ethnographic work included here ultimately seeks to value our perspectives of health and mental health, placing culture and place at the core of getting well and staying well. For Tom and myself, it is our hope that we begin a dialogue that promotes respect, value, and an understanding about the people of the southern Appalachian region. We hope to further and deepen the understanding of the culture of Cherokee people.

For Tom, "One has to first understand how that culture views what everyone else looks at. The only way to do that effectively is to get those concepts linguistically. How does the language interpret the world for people of Appalachia and Cherokee? It is based on our knowledge and experience of that world. The broadening of that perspective of how the world works and what it means spawns wisdom. It's not to exclude the expanding of that understanding, but it leads to wisdom. When you read it, it's a window in understanding an older way and practice of how lives were lived." He continues,

> The things that Cherokee consider sacred manifest themselves in our language, our songs and symbolism. These are manifested in sounds, and in the meaning of those sounds, and in the symbolism of what is sacred and meaningful. The songs and even the things we wore were heard and seen by the observer, they would understand who we were by these things. This book is a representation of an age-old way of doing things. It is a product of our language. It is our song, as sacred as water; it is our symbols manifested in wood, shell, and clay, in gorgets, baskets, and pottery. This is how we communicated. If that is what you present, it is sacred—our word is sacred or should be if it is to mean anything. It is to present and then see the relevance of our concept of how things in the world work or function in the right way, or *duyuk'dv'i* [this spelling matches pronunciation; the spelling *duyugodv'i* corresponds with the grammatically correct syllabary; see table I.1]. It's like water, it becomes something living, animate. To continue to speak about these things, they stay alive. They are living, they are sacred. The sounds of the language—the ups and downs and breath—make it real. With this language you make it sacred. It lives inside of you. It guides you. Dead things can't make sounds. It must continue to be spoken and heard. It is our song.

TABLE I.1. CHEROKEE SYLLABARY

a	e	i	o	u	v
D a	R e	T i	Ꮉ o	Oʼ u	i v
Ꮝ Ꮵ ga ka	Ᏼ ge / ke	y gi / ki	A go / ko	J gu / ku	E gv / kv
Ꮀ ha	Ꮄ he	Ꮂ hi	Ᏺ ho	Γ hu	Ꮔ hv
W la	Ꮅ le	Ꮈ li	G lo	M lu	Ꮃ lv
Ꮄ ma	Ol me	H mi	Ꮎ mo	y mu	Ꮇ mv
Θ Ꮏ G na hna nah	Ꮑ ne	h ni	Z no	Ꮅ nu	Oʋ nv
Ᏻ gwa / qua	Ꮶ gwe / que	Ꮲ gwi / qui	Ꮵ° gwo / quo	Ꮹ gwu / quu	Ɛ gwv / quv
Ᏸ Ꮝ sa s	4 se	b si	Ꮊ so	Ꮪ su	R sv
Ꮭ da / ta	Sꚋ de te	ᎫᎫ di ti	V do / to	S du / tu	Ꮯ° dv / tv
Ꮧ Ꮧ dla tla	L dle	C dli	Ꮴ dlo	Ꮻ dlu	P dlv
W tsa	V tse	Ᏺ tsi	K tso	Ꮪ tsu	Cͦ tsv
G wa	Ꮾ we	Θ wi	Ꮼ wo	9 wu	6 wv
Ꮿ ya	ß ya	Ꮽ yi	ᏸ yo	Gͦ yu	B ya

Source: Thomas N. Belt.

Literary great N. Scott Momaday (Kiowa) provides an example of that connectedness. He did not have to walk on that ground his whole life, but he was told about the Kiowa homeland, and the language conveyed the life that existed for his father and grandparents. The truth and reality of the language was spoken, and it made home in his heart and his soul. It is the sound of well-being, of being a whole person and getting place to be our reality of who we are. The stories and the language teach us of the relationships between us and the trees and the landscape and the animals and the water and all that is a part of us. To others it is only myth or stories or folklore, but to the people who speak this language, it brings life to things that supposedly are dead or appear to be unconnected. It brings relationships to an existence that, to the larger society, doesn't exist or at the very least is unimportant. The key to these relationships is the interconnection between us all. For Tom, "These words become sacred, important. English is sometimes just labels. These words aren't a code for English. They represent an understanding of relationships and connections that are thousands and maybe millions of years old."

To quote Momaday (1988), "There is great good in returning to a landscape that has had extraordinary meaning in one's life. It happens that we return to such places in our minds irresistibly. There are certain villages and towns, mountains and plains that, having seen them walked in them lived in them even for a day, we keep forever in the mind's eye. They become indispensable to our well-being; they define us, and we say: I am who I am because I have been there, or there."

In chapter 1, we introduce readers to cultural concepts of health (*tohi*), and Tom discusses connected, essential ideas that place language at the center of the Cherokee worldview regarding health, science, and behavior. Tom shares linguistically how Kituwah people make sense of the world around them via the cultural concept of *du-yu-go-dv-i* (SGA6'T), which influences their understanding of behavior, natural laws, and life lived as a "real human being," all critical in being whole and healthy. The wisdom of these concepts is understood as they have been handed down through language use generationally for thousands of years.

As we are interested in health for individuals, we also posit that the healing of Indigenous communities must be involved to secure the success of members' well-being. We emphasize the need for Indigenous women of these communities—part of a matrilineal tribal nation—to regain their roles as nurturers, healers, and leaders to foster community healing. After Contact (1500 CE), the traditional roles of both men and women began a process of rapid change. Because women reflected the stability and organization of the community and provided the identity for all members, I would go as far as to say that without the subjugation of Native women, colonization could not have happened. This has detrimentally affected Native communities generationally. In order for communities to heal, their women must be respected, and their medicine, childbirth, and child-rearing must be addressed. Chapter 2, we hope, will generate more dialogue about how to support women in Indigenous communities to restore *tohi*.

Throughout this book, we rely on the preservation of traditional knowledge, or Native science, via the language to provide insight as to why we should recognize our connection to the land. These notions are supported through a variety of disciplines and examples. Chapter 3 underscores the value and importance of traditional knowledge that has been handed down for millennia through the language of Native peoples. Citing the wisdom and insight of Native scholars such as Vine Deloria Jr. and Dawn Martin-Hill, we see a critical component of the Indigenous paradigm: "connectivity" and the importance of relationships that are reflected in the landscape and teaching of what is "natural law."

Chapter 4 discusses the importance of cosmography, the cultural and historical significance of the landscape. In this chapter several specific sites and historical figures are examined to exemplify the critical nature of site preservation and natural resources, and the ways these help in providing identity of people to place. As the land base for Native peoples was greatly reduced, lost, or changed, it had a direct impact on their awareness of who they were as a people. We suggest that now more than ever, recognition of historical sites and homeland boundaries proves essential for a healthy self-concept and understanding of identity as a people and nation.

Again, we consider the importance of language in preserving the Native science and traditional knowledge to help people be *tohi*. Chapter 5 concerns Indigenous approaches to counseling. In my work with tribal agencies regarding health and mental issues, it occurred to me to ask about how certain topics may have been perceived linguistically by Kituwah people. I began by asking speakers how to say something in Cherokee, and then asking them to translate that back into English. Each time, a new way of looking at an issue was gained, one that broadened the meaning and understanding and could be beneficial to health professionals working with the community. When I worked with Native youth, I witnessed the ethnocentrism inherent in behavioral services and sought to learn more about how culture heals and resonates better in providing services for Native people. In teaching a course on Indigenous and Western psychologies, I have had the privilege of meeting and learning from several Native psychologists who have been urging Indigenous communities to develop their own culturally based treatment approaches. Tom, who also has worked with Native youth, was key in contributing Kituwah-specific language and processes in potential counseling approaches.

Chapter 6 looks at how subjugation of Indigenous knowledge since Contact has impeded the benefit of that understanding for everyone. It has only been in recent years that Western science has promoted research that acknowledges the wisdom and early achievements of Indigenous communities. In this chapter Tom provides examples of how Kituwah language is a science-based language that helps explain the dynamics of the world around us. Physicists such as David Bohm have integrated the traditional knowledge of Native people into their work, highlighting its importance. Other disciplines in medicine, botany, and biology that historically siloed their work are more and more recognizing the importance of interdisciplinary research and the interconnectedness of our life and relationships. As we see the bigger picture of how all is related, it becomes clearer how we affect one another through our behaviors and beliefs about how things work.

Chapter 7 reiterates the need to consider "decolonizing"—or, more appropriately, "Indigenizing"—the way we live and perceive the world. As is important in societies that value everyone's contributions and worth, the emphasis is placed on our connection to one another and to the natural world. With impending, serious damage as a result of climate change, for example, it is imperative that we shift our thinking not just on ourselves but on our actions, and consider how they can be of value to the overall effort to lessen the stress on our environment. We witness the devasting fires, colossal rains, and winds of storms in our country and around the world, the warming of glacial waters, the cost of human and animal lives; we must recognize it as a way of living, of consuming, and of producing that can have a tremendous impact on how our future will be realized for generations soon to come. Michael Yellow Bird's work to have us be more mindful of our connections to our food sources and our relationships with others harks back to those cultural values of service and honor to others. Making time to assess our lives and worldview can improve the quality of life not only for ourselves but for others. There was a way in which Kituwahs navigated their landscape that reflected this way of thinking, to live our lives in full understanding of how we touch all else around us.

Also, for many Appalachian people, their souls lie in the soil and altitude of ridgelines and mountainsides. The streams and rivers bring a solitude and comfort that they will always be here as they always have. In the rapidly changing culture, loss of dialect, loss of an agrarian lifeway, loss of a manner of socializing, we have comfort that the mountains and the creatures that reside there should remain. We share our love for this place with the first inhabitants and have learned from them the healing that can come from just being here. A wonderful, edited volume by Jessica Cory entitled *Mountains Piled upon Mountains* (2019) contains the writings of more than fifty contributors, bringing their awe, love, and respect for Appalachia's natural world. As renowned Appalachian writer Mae Claxton mentions early on, "every Appalachian writer is an environmentalist" (1). Early explorers, settlers, historians, writers, and Indigenous leaders have written about the beauty and spectacular wonders of Appalachia, but little about the ways their beliefs and worldviews intertwine.

In reviewing the literature regarding Appalachian and Native relations, perspectives, and symbiosis, the record is scant. The distinguished North Carolina historian Hugh Talmage Lefler used to be *the* source of learning about the people of the Tar Heel state. He authored or coauthored many years of North Carolina history textbooks for public schools (usually seventh grade), and if young mountain people were looking for that section that talked about our part of the state, western North Carolina, they were in for a grave disappointment. Very little was ever mentioned about the region or the Cherokee people, even though the Cherokee people had lived in that area for millennia, and most people who came to western North Carolina came to visit the Cherokee.

A 1954 text that Lefler coauthored with Albert Ray Newsome has all of four pages about "the Indians of North Carolina" and not surprisingly speaks mostly about those tribes in the piedmont and coastal areas of the state, all of which they say have "disappeared" except for the Cherokee, which they mention only a few times, it seems in passing. As for the Appalachian region, equally little attention is paid. For those of us attending public schools, then, it is little wonder that what is known about the people, history, and culture of the region must be garnered by listening to our own folks share about life in the mountains. Unfortunately, that leaves most people to rely on other sources for their understanding about how people lived here and what the realities of their lives have been.

It is undeniable that early settlers into the Appalachian region took advantage of land speculation and other means of possession to take land from the original inhabitants of the southern Appalachian region. A tremendous amount of violence and death via wars, homicides, disease, and other traumas of injustice were committed. In a 1957 article, Henry T. Malone mildly portrays this often violent and chaotic transformation:

> The early nineteenth century was a period of tremendous adjustment for the Cherokees, an era characterized by contrasting relationships with white men. The belligerent, relentless push of pioneers, the infiltration of friendly traders and artisans, and the constructive guidance of able Indian agents and missionaries made inevitable far-reaching changes in both Cherokee mores and relations with the whites. After a crippling defeat by American forces in the Revolutionary War, the Cherokees were slowly confined by a series of treaties into a tightly encircled area in the southern Appalachians. Forced into a new type of existence by sharply reduced hunting grounds and exposed to the more comfortable agrarian economy of the white man through the example and teaching of traders and Indian agents, the tribe began a change in its pattern of life. (1)

Malone further notes that "this occurred despite the efforts of some white men to destroy that security through theft, persuasion, treaty, or the illegal. Thus to the early nineteenth-century Cherokee white man appeared as a paradox—offering both friendship and hostility, guidance and abandonment, inspiration and degradation" (14).

We cannot ignore that our histories intersect. Too little has been recorded of the sharing and friendship that has been exchanged among these mountain families. It is unrealistic to think that occupation of non-Native families in Southern Appalachia for close to three hundred years has not been without symbiotic exchange. We hope that this work illuminates the friendship and optimism we have shared with one another, provides a clear example of our learning from one another, and highlights the positives rather than the stereotypes that have dominated our more recent histories. Our language, culture, and worldview have meaning and value. We know who we are because of these things. They make us whole.

Chapter One

‹‹‹‹‹‹‹‹‹‹‹‹‹‹‹‹‹‹‹‹‹‹‹‹‹‹‹‹‹

TOHI (Ꮣ)

Connection is health. And what our society
does its best to disguise from us is how ordinary,
how commonly attainable, health is.

WENDELL BERRY

Tohi (pronounced tow hee) is the Kituwah word for health. This word's popular use was revived after a meeting of elders and clinicians in Cherokee several years ago. Thomas N. Belt was asked to help translate for the Cherokee-
language speakers there, most of whom were elders, and he explained for the
majority of attendees who were not Cherokee speakers what *tohi* meant. Immediately thereafter, the health and medical community there began to use
the term often, and it has become fairly commonly used as a substitute for
the English word "health."

Revitalizing Cherokee language is always a step in the right direction, including this example, but, unfortunately, substituting a Cherokee word for
an English word isn't sufficient for fully realizing the importance of the language. In Tom's words, language *is* medicine. It is health. Tom elaborates:

> There is a disconnect between providers and people who need help. Health
> becomes dispensary. In other words, come to me and I'll give you some-
> thing. This thing is what you need, not me but this thing. The help is dis-
> pensing what you need. That becomes a business. In our way, the way to il-
> lustrate healing is, you need a house, right? I have tools, I have some things
> that you can use to build that house with and you don't have that right now.
> So, I'm just not going to give you those tools, that material. You and I are
> going to build this house. We're going to be in it together. I'm going to do
> just as much work as you are. And in doing that you and I become con-
> nected, we depend on each other, we understand the importance of what

we're doing, the things we have, and in the end then we complete this structure, and you can live in it and you'll be safe. But we did this together. Without that, if I just tossed the stuff out there, you may never get it done without anybody helping. You won't be safe. If there's no one there to help you, you won't achieve that healing and things won't ever get better unless I'm involved in it. It makes the effort stronger, more effective . . . all those things that are attributed to doing something right, to being successful. It's putting things in the right order. When you say you need my help, when you come to me for help, or when you go to one of those people for help, they will join you in that effort. They won't take on that thing without you. That house isn't for me, it's for you, but I'll do everything I can to help. We'll get it done. It's the best way to do it. Wouldn't you consider that the most scientific, or logical, way to do it? Rather than being just a dispensary source, you become an engaged participant in the healing process. That is the way we looked at the health aspect of people, we all had to help. We've talked about how sometimes healers had to bring in other healers to help. They understood the importance of communal work. They didn't overlook the fact that the more hands helping was better than trying to do something yourself. Unfortunately, there are some who do for self-aggrandizement or for people to take pity, or for ego, and it serves no purpose. We have to understand that it takes everybody. To try to do something yourself is not *duyuk'dv'i* (SGAᎤ°T, the right or correct path).

Tom also emphasizes the language in use of medicine. He says,

But we also have our own voices. The sound of our voices, in terms of songs and sacred formulas, these words that we use and things we say were determined a long time ago. They emit a specific sound that makes healing conducive. It has to be heard. If you don't hear a train coming, you're out of luck. You have to hear your child crying, you have to hear what they have to say, you have to hear your relatives speak, before you can help them. It communicates needs, but voice also communicates giving of healing. That's why we have songs to heal. Trees even make sound. Languages were specific to the geographic area where people lived. The way older Cherokee women spoke, a singsong lower tone, always reminded me of the sound of water going over rocks. It was melodious and flowing. Language replicated the environment. The sounds of birds and water. The importance was to fit in with everything around you. The sacred songs were part of that connecting with the environment and helped us to understand how to live here.

We speak mountain talk, and we know exactly what that is and where it is from. You have to conduct yourself in a way that is appropriate to where you live, and to speak the same. It communicates where you're from and where you live. *You are of a place, and not just from it.* Europeans who came here quickly became mountain people. Speaking of his talks with my mother, Tom says,

> From what your mom said, these mountains are the fabric of her being. She was of this place. Sounds of being here are healing. Getting closer to *duyuk'dv'i* is getting closer to healing and being whole. Connection to place is medicine. Just like a mother's voice connects her child to her. The sound is a conduit for reconnecting and healing. These are the sounds of *tohi*. It becomes medicine. Ceremonies, words, and songs are born of the very dirt or ground we live on. We consider that a scientific fact. That's why language is so important. It's not just for an exchange of ideas, but language is more than that. Stories from our elders recall that our language was sacred, speech was sacred. It could be used to heal. Conversely it can be used to harm. It's just a sound, right? But we all know that language can hurt. The Kituwah way is to use language to heal, and it reflects living a life on the right path, *duyuk'dv'i*, the right way, the right path. Use your voice for the right purpose, to help people when they are lost or hurting. The saying of words in ceremony, if used in the right way, is a way to heal, to put you back on that right road. We want you to have a good life, to be healthy.

So *tohi*, in the Kituwah world, reflects things moving in a normal, peaceful way. "Elders have described *tohi* as the clouds and grass moving at their own pace, not rushed or urgent. There is a fluidness to life. Harmony and well-being, balance and peace, can reflect the essence of *tohi*. Illness, harmfulness, stress can pull one away from *tohi*, particularly if left to be dealt with for any length of time."

Most English speakers usually refer to health as the absence of disease and do not think deeper about peace equating with health. For Kituwahs, peace, health, or *tohi* can also come from the idea of having a clear conscience. A state of being *tohi* is more than just a word list. The concept of *tohi* infers a more pervasive understanding that the relationships in your life are all balanced and moving forward in a good way. Making good choices and having good relationships are inclusive in the understanding that you are connected and upright, moving forward and looking out for others. If we are stressing out in our own lives, very little can be left to do for others. Our energy and focus are on ourselves, and the normal flow is disrupted.

To be out of *tohi* is to be out of balance. As Heidi M. Altman and Belt (2009) discuss, "In examining the occurrence of illness in the Cherokee view, it is necessary first to understand that within the category of illness or imbalance an individual can have experiences related to his or her own actions, or those related to the actions of someone else, either of which can disrupt their own ongoing fluidity or push them out of their proper state of neutrality" (19). Those helping return one back to balance may try to get a broad understanding of what has been going on with the "patient" and ask general questions about what has been happening in their world without talking about pain or listing physical ailments. The understanding is that past regressions, transgressions, malice, or hard feelings can upset the balance of a relationship and eventually manifest in illness.

It is the belief of Kituwahs that the manifestation of words and sounds has purpose in the principles of living well. They describe scientific concepts learned from thousands of years of observing, studying, and learning how things happen and are connected. The importance of words and their construction is exemplified in the word at the core of this manuscript, *tohi*. *Tohi* carries the two sounds—long *o* and long *e*—that indicate the habitual aspect of Cherokee words. These two sounds designate the concept of eternalness or perpetuity. For example, *o* and *e* (*o*, *i* in Cherokee) can be added to any verb to make it perpetual. To Cherokees that means "it exists" or "it is real" or it is "a reality." When you make it a real thing it is part of creation. In perspective of dealing with the importance of something being "a real thing" or *udohiyu* (closely related to *tohi*), it means you can't just talk with someone or punish them, you have to deal with them in a real way that makes connecting them to the larger understanding of who you are important. *Udohiyu*, true reality, acknowledges it is more than an opinion but is rather a real issue or habitual behavior. It is more than just a judgment passed; it depicts an issue that is real. An illustration of this is *a di tas go i* (ᎠᏗᏘᏍᎪᎢ), which means he/she always drinks (is an alcoholic/alcoholism). Drinking, then, is an identifier of who that person is, but it is where they are on their path, not their identity. In a traditional way, it, much like disease, is viewed as an entity that comes to visit. In this way, when a behavior becomes problematic, it is an anomalous visitor that must be dealt with if it is to leave. This way of thinking isn't about being critical of the person; it is about identifying a behavior that must be addressed because you must be in balance to be *tohi*. Ultimately, the language reflects that the person is redeemable and can be assisted in finding their way back on the right path or *duyuk'dv'i*, directing them to *tohi*.

Tohi can mean wellness or peace, moving at one's own pace or moving at one's own speed. It means being unstressed or unforced. This is particularly applicable to the discussion of the prevention and/or maintenance of diabetes. Moving at your own pace, walking at your own speed is good exercise. Being unstressed is a major issue in understanding diabetes and chronic disease: "Reducing toxic stress can target the common physiologic pathway implicated in an enormous array of health outcomes from asthma to cardio-vascular disease" (Johnson et al. 2013, 325).

The impact of chronic stress and disease was well understood in Indian country for a couple of decades prior to the more generalized understanding of this connection in other communities. The impact of historical and inter-generational trauma was a model first introduced by psychoanalyst Eva Fo-gelman, who conducted research among Holocaust survivors and their chil-dren. Her work in this field led her and her colleagues to train other mental health professionals extensively in the treatment of individuals who have suf-fered massive historical trauma, including Native American populations.

From these early beginnings, social scientists, counselors, physicians, and other health professionals have brought their work together to move for-ward an understanding of the intersection of biology and environment. Epi-genetics, which is exemplary of this intersecting science, allows us to under-stand the long-term implications of historical and intergenerational trauma, adverse childhood experiences, chronic stress, and chronic disease. Epi-genetics is defined as the "study of changes in organisms caused by modi-fication of gene expression rather than alteration of the genetic code itself" (Oxford University Press, n.d., s.v. "epigenetics"). We understand better how genes can be turned on or off by environmental factors, which can have a di-rect impact on health, not only for ourselves but for future generations.

More recently Native scholars are using the knowledge of these models to discuss more culturally appropriate ways with which to address stress and trauma issues. Joseph P. Gone and Eduardo Duran, for instance, have advo-cated for use of language, culture, and ceremony to help heal.

For Cherokees, the strategy to address this includes cultural models that involve ceremony and the first element of being Kituwah: *gadugi* (ᏍᏏᏴ, mak-ing oneself available to serve others). This means making opportunities to spend time with others and to develop an identity centered in service. Some-times this means coming clean; you cannot be accessible to ceremony if you are "using." It is taking the obligation of service as a Kituwah person seri-ously and making that one's reality.

Tom relayed a story of a man who was an alcoholic and decided to go to a medicine person for help. The elder told him that he would help him but that he needed to attend ceremony, but it would be held in a year and he was to come back. In the meantime, he was told to spend his next year serving others. So, he began to go to others and see whether they needed him to help them with cutting wood and any other tasks. As the days went by he realized that the more he served, the less he drank. A year passed, and the man went back to the medicine man. The elder asked whether he had been drinking, and the man said, "No, I've been getting to know people and being a part of my community." "Good," said the elder. "You are ready for ceremony."

My mother had a book on medicine entitled *Gunn's Domestic Medicine*, originally published in 1830. This book had been passed down in her family for generations. It was a medical manual for those living in remote areas who couldn't access a physician. It contained detailed information on everything from amputations, to bloodletting, to treatments for the clap. The last portion of the book contained descriptions of many plant medicinals and their usages, and in the first portion of the book was a rather lengthy discussion of how one's emotions affected health. Not unlike Kituwahs, this early practitioner understood the value of people acknowledging and identifying their emotions as a direct connection with health.

Volumes could be written about *tohi*, but it is better understood by those who have the gift of the Cherokee language and the cultural contexts in which that language and accompanying songs should be used. This text will provide only a glimpse into these ancient paradigms regarding health and hopefully provide examples that are of benefit to those interested in a healthy life. Tom hopes that even though these are not definitive and exhaustive discussions, they still may prove helpful and reflect the need for and urgency of language preservation.

Chapter Two

MAKING A CONNECTION BETWEEN INDIGENOUS WOMEN, HISTORY, AND HEALING THE COMMUNITY

A Brief Introduction to Matrilineality

> Cherokee is our check-cashing name. Our real name is Kituwah, People of the soil that belongs to the Creator.
>
> THOMAS N. BELT

Probably the most well-known Native tribe in the world is the Cherokee. What many do not realize is there are only three Cherokee tribes that are federally recognized: the United Keetoowah Band and the Cherokee Nation, both in Oklahoma, and the Eastern Band of Cherokee Indians (EBCI), located in their collective and shared homeland of western North Carolina. They each have the same ancient history, and all originated from what is now known as the sacred mother town of Kituwah in western North Carolina. Here they lived for more than twelve thousand years in parts of states today known as North Carolina, Tennessee, Virginia, Kentucky, South Carolina, Georgia, and Alabama.

In Tom's keynote address at the 2019 Rooted in the Mountains Symposium, he said:

> The purpose of Rooted in the Mountains has, for the last ten years, been to educate and highlight the substance of life in these mountains. The substance of who we are, the things that make life here possible, the things that make life here incredibly diverse and different from any place else that I've ever lived. It's to showcase life in these mountains. The age of these mountains and the tremendous biological diversity provide a legacy for those who live here. We live in a place that is both ancient and profoundly diverse. . . .

Connection to this very old place and a deeply intrinsic connection is reflected in living here for over thirteen millennia. In that time we had a system of understanding that reflected stewardship. Social, political, and religious aspects of our society, as well as the birth of our language, are absolute reflections of connection to this place. Even through the spoken word, through the way our words were used, this was a reflection of these mountains. What we learned about it coincided with what we learned about having to live here, being in these mountains. . . . This understanding, this science of living here, even gave us our name. Cherokee is not even a Cherokee word. It is what others called us. The real name we call ourselves is the word Kituwah from the word *Otsigiduwagi* (ᏍᎯᏴᏍᎬᏴ)—we are the people of the Kituwah.

Their place of origin, Kituwah, is considered a sacred "mother town." The earth is considered the female that supports all life and is imbued with diversity and mystery of which all is yet to be understood. It is Kanane'ski Amayi ehi (ᎦᎾᏟᏍᎠᏴ ᎠᏔᎶ Ꭱ.Ꮝ, Grandmother Water Spider), an essential being in the Kituwah creation story, who weaved her web into a bowl on her back and brought to the people the fire unattainable by all others who had tried. Selu (ᏎᎷ, the Corn Mother), a central figure in the provision of food, and the Sun, a female entity that provides light and warmth, again are crucial to the existence of the Kituwah people. But one of my more recent conversations with Tom was exceptionally revealing regarding the cultural and historical status of women in Kituwah society. Their particular shell gorget (necklace) motif is fairly well known and attributed to important Mississippian-era material culture for southeastern tribes, including Kituwahs (figure 2.1). This figure has a four-sided design with the head of a woodpecker on each of the four sides, which I had always regarded as a motif of warriors, but as Tom spoke of the design, he (and students from Stanford University in his Cherokee-language class) began to understand this as a pervasive symbol of life itself. The language and meaning were symbiotic with water, the life-giving element for all living things, and, correspondingly, were symbiotic with women, also life giving.

Tom explained, "The cross in the middle is the fire of Kituwah. Kituwah is what is around the fire. The four sides are both a water symbol and *duyckti duyuk'dv'i* (the right way or path). These encircle Kituwah and our world. The woodpeckers are the protectors of our world. There is land because this was brought up from the beetle and spider, both of whom are female—she brought the fire. We correlate these important elements with matrilineality. The symbols placed on these gorgets reflect how we are supposed to think. People think of 'mother nature' and rightly so because nature is effeminate as it gives birth and rebirth. You have to know these things in order to be connected."

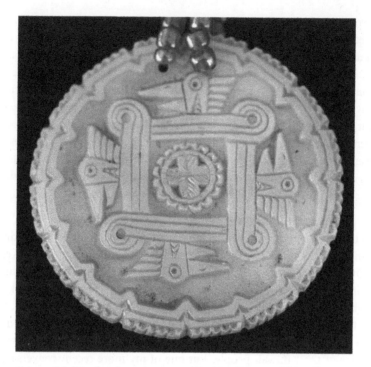

FIGURE 2.1. Woodpecker gorget carved by Dan Townsend (Creek).
Courtesy of Rosemary Peek.

With this understanding, I had always wondered why James Mooney,
one of the most famous ethnographers who worked with the Cherokee at
the turn of the twentieth century, referred to rivers—critical water sources in
Cherokee territory—as "the Long Man." It seemed to contradict the association of women with all other sources of life, if indeed rivers were considered
to be masculine. So I asked Tom about this, and in normal fashion, he responded linguistically, "Mooney made an assumption based on his standard
of reference as a man during the Victorian era, and translated rivers as *gah
nuh hee dah* (long) *a sga ya* (man), when in fact, it should have been translated *gah nuh hee dah* (long) *yuh wee* (person/human) (ᏴᎾ ᏐᎤᏫ)." This
had bothered me for a long time, and finally it made sense.

These and other female references support the centrality and critical importance of women in Kituwah society, which, like most tribes first exposed
to Europeans, was matrilineal. Kituwah women wielded great responsibilities for their people. One's identity as a Kituwah person, or human being,
came from one source, one's biological mother. The importance of women
to the civil, social, and cultural integrity of Indigenous peoples cannot be

overstated. Europeans could not have colonized the New World without destroying the position and status of women. Therefore, the long journey of healing these communities will not come fully until their positions of respect and honor have returned.

In addition, those who today would be considered "alternative gendered," or LGBTQ, traditionally had an important place in Cherokee and other tribal societies. Historian Peter Wood (1992) writes:

> Most Indians, including those in the South, recognized androgynous men known as berdaches who dressed as women and accepted non-masculine roles. Far from despising the berdaches, Indians respected them for sharing male and female traits and often granted them important ceremonial status. But by the era of Columbus, the fear of homosexuality had grown into a powerful force in Christian Europe, and suppression of sexual diversity was especially intense in Spain. When [Spanish explorer Pedro] Menendez pressed for permission to expand the slave trade from Florida, he accused local chiefs of [being] "infamous people, Sodomites." He explained to the King of Spain, "it would greatly serve God Our Lord and your Majesty if these same were dead, or given as slaves." (25)

Wood wrote this at a time when the term *berdache* was still used in historical sources and academic circles. Since then, there has been slow yet important movement in research among American Indian and Alaska Native populations as well as other Indigenous communities to understand more about the cultural context and significance of alternative gendered people.

Gregory D. Smithers makes a rare foray into this topic in a 2014 article on Cherokee "two spirits." Other scholars, particularly since the 1980s, such as Walter L. Williams, Sabine Lang, Will Roscoe, Brian Joseph Gilley, Gilbert Herdt, Sue-Ellen Jacobs, Wesley Thomas, and Lester B. Brown, have researched the variety, place, and social status of these individuals among Indigenous people. A consensus has emerged that an underlying rationale for such an acceptable spectrum of gender identity is that Creator doesn't make mistakes and we all have purpose. Discussing this topic for Kituwah people many years ago, Tom relayed a moving story about someone who was known and loved in his community for his kindness and service to others, a person who was referred to as *ta li tsu da na do gi* (ᏔᎵ ᏧᏓᎾᏙᎩ) or, as Tom translated, a person of "two hearts." He said he could also be called *ta li u da na do i tsu we hv i* (ᏔᎵ ᎤᏓᎾᏙᎢ ᏧᏪᎲᎢ, two souls or things that have consciousness living in them), another beautiful thought. The place of those who are alternative gendered or have the spirit and heart of both men and women as part of the natural world is reflected in both the animal and plant worlds as well.

Because these people were often the first terminated in the colonial inva-sion, much of their history was destroyed. However, their place in tribal soci-eties was still noted in early sketches or briefly mentioned in travel memoirs in Indian country. This is apparent in references as diverse as Cherokee men who historically "assumed the dress and performed all the duties of women and who lived their whole life in this manner" (Smithers 2014, 628) and the more recent observations of men shaking shells at spiritual gatherings, tra-ditionally a woman's role (Driskill 2008). Most well known and documented were "war women" who courageously went to battle with men in the era of revolution, today echoed in references to women playing stickball, "little brother of war" or more appropriately "little sister of war." Each example re-flects the important social and cultural roles of Kituwah people, male and fe-male, and more hopefully their continued place in contemporary society will not go unnoticed and unappreciated.

Mohawk elder Katsi Cook (2012) advocates the idea that women are the first environment for everyone. She refers often in her talks to "layered envi-ronments of meaning of the Indigenous woman's body: (1) cosmological—bodies shaped by the logic of cosmology or having cosmological meaning in origin teachings; (2) mythological—restoration of sacred knowledge, ceremony, and symbolic narratives; (3) territorial—ecosystems, metaphors of body and landscapes; (4) historical—impact of 'Doctrine of Discovery' and the resulting efforts to recover, decolonize, and heal; (5) sociological—kinship, identity, and ritual; and (6) biological—evolution, epigenetics, psycho-neuroimmunology." These paradigms are diametrically opposed to Western society's ideas of women's bodies and even of the natural event of birthing, which has been medicalized and, as Cook says, "couched in fear."

Millennia-long life in societies holding women central in their governance and position miraculously left vestiges of their sacredness even after almost total eradication of Native peoples. Cook (2012) speaks to Indigenous women, telling them they must "come out of silence and use their voices to reconstruct their tradition . . . women's empowerment is grounded in knowledge of the body." Another residual of colonization is that when violence is perpetuated against women, a common response is to become psychologically numb and more dissociated with one's own body, antithetical to traditional empower-ment. These are issues unfortunately common today. According to a recent review article, "Various national and regional studies have found that violence against women is more widespread and severe among self-identified AI/AN [American Indian and Alaska Native] people than among other North Amer-ican people," and they "were significantly more likely than women from all other backgrounds to have been raped and/or stalked at some point in their lifetime" (Crossland, Palmer, and Brooks 2013, 772–73).

The subjugation of Cherokee women began soon after the arrival of Europeans. For Cherokees, the long and complicated history from Contact (around 1500 CE) up to 1835 reflects tremendous, rapid change that wreaked havoc on their way of life. Wars, disease, colonization, assimilation, exploitation, discrimination, and attempted termination instigated trauma and change in every aspect of living, thinking, and believing.

To exemplify just how pervasive the assimilation and cultural changes were, Cherokee studies scholar William G. McLoughlin (1986) reflects on six areas of "cultural transformation" experienced by the Cherokees, beginning with the shifting roles and responsibilities of women. He organized these changes as: (1) a transformation in familial roles and kinship—a movement from a matrilineal, exogamous (marrying outside the group) clan system to a more patriarchal, nuclear family system, and from communal cooperation (*gadugi*) to individualism; (2) economic transformation—from fur trading and bartering to federal policy–directed programs of agriculture and a cash economy; (3) social and ethical transformations—a decline of the "harmony ethic" or hospitality ethics and movement toward the accumulation of wealth through inheritance via lineages, and eventually the development of socioeconomic stratification and distinctions that would be made via education in white schools; (4) political transformation—disregard for the place of clan membership in civil responsibilities (with each town historically being self-sufficient and self-governing, and women having prominence in the council houses), centralization of government and authority, and the adoption of an elective, bicameral legislative system with courts, police, and so forth; (5) religious transformation—a movement from pluralism to an adaptation of a monotheistic, Christian theology, which also reinforced shifts in cultural values (e.g., compartmentalized religiosity in place of permeating spirituality); and (6) a transformation from an oral to written tradition. For many, this last transformation began after Sequoyah's creation of the syllabary around 1823, which also promoted socialization and shifts in teaching approaches.

What is miraculous is that Cherokee society is still living and thriving today. I've heard people, even in North Carolina, who believed all Indians to be dead. It is somewhat understandable that most people lack knowledge of American Indian history, even though it is a critical part of our history. As a former teacher of history and lecturer in Native studies, I have seen over and over again that American history has failed us. The truth about death, trauma, and attempted elimination of the "Indian problem" by government policies and agencies wasn't successfully taught in our school systems. Despite my being an avid and interested student of history, the incomplete and intentionally misleading early history of the Indigenous people of the western hemisphere was the only offering I encountered. Not until graduate school did the truth about our dysfunctional and catastrophic relationship with Indigenous people become clear to me.

Today, more primary documents of that early clash of cultures and more scholarly texts by Native peoples themselves are available, but unfortunately most students do not avail themselves of Native studies literature or even have the opportunity to discover it. Previously, very little in the media or literature presented the reality of how Native people navigated and adapted to the rapidly changing and dangerous world that the colonizers brought to them. However, in recent years there appears to be more interest in the truths regarding the making of our country, and in the diversity of those who were made to suffer through it.

The Cherokee people are often some of the first to come to mind when Indigenous people in the United States are discussed, perhaps because of their numbers or because of the historic "Trail of Tears," but hopefully more for their resilience and progressive vision for overcoming adversity and being successful in dealing with their challenges. In Gregory D. Smithers's *The Cherokee Diaspora* (2015), a better understanding of how Cherokee people migrated and sought to create new lives in the face of discrimination, poverty, and uncertainty becomes clear. Smithers provides a good overview of origins and movements, though overlooking some of the earlier population reduction efforts, such as those that targeted the Cherokee Lower Towns. However, Thomas M. Hatley's *Dividing Paths* (1995) can provide students an understanding of the stark changes that affected and eradicated these towns by the end of the revolutionary era.

It was clear even by 1745 that Cherokee leaders were gravely concerned by how quickly they had become dependent on the newcomers. Chief Skegunsta made a plea to the governor of South Carolina: "I . . . have always told my people to be well with the English for they cannot expect any supply from any where else, nor can they live independent of the English. What are we red people? The clothes we wear, we cannot make ourselves. They are made [for] us. We use their ammunition with which to kill deer. We cannot make our guns, they are made [for] us. Every necessary thing in life we must have from the white people" (McDowell 1958, 453).

Inferior trade goods were often foisted on Natives so that they would have to come back more often for replacements, keeping tribes locked into trade relationships. Distilled alcohol, introduced by Europeans, was considered a main element in trade with tribal nations. As a result, indulgent drinking was often encouraged as well as modeled by Europeans as a means to facilitate unfair trade and outright theft of goods. As historian Francis Paul Prucha (1984) has stated, "the fundamental policy of Indian Affairs was to make the Indians dependent on the English in their trade" (8).

Nevertheless, after more than five centuries of colonization and assimilation, Cherokee families held on to their identity as Natives, even though some migrated into other parts of the world. Smithers (2015) estimates that over one million people throughout the globe identify their ancestry from Cherokees.

Hundreds of groups call themselves Cherokee, yet only the three aforementioned "official" tribes have that two-edged sword of federal recognition. Federal recognition status means clear delineation from all the thousands of others who identify themselves as Cherokee descendants. Those who are formally enrolled in one of the three Cherokee nations have afforded to them all rights and privileges of being tribal citizens, including access to the treaty-promised services unique to tribal nations. This status comes from generations of survival and resiliency in the face of unsurmountable odds of eradication. They have earned their rights and heritage by successfully overcoming discrimination encoded in Indian policies over two hundred years, and surviving the outright efforts of elimination.

These three Cherokee nations have had to hide, move, resettle, and reconstruct their societies under great threat. They are now three separate political entities, each dealing with its own legal and civil battles in its own region. When the United Keetoowahs and the Cherokee Nation ancestors went west to Indian Territory, it was stated by the leadership who remained in North Carolina that they forfeited their claim to their homeland, even if they left under duress. In John R. Finger's *The Eastern Band of Cherokees, 1819–1900* (1984), the long and complicated issues of tribal factionalism, the pursuit of citizenship in North Carolina, and the back-and-forth migration between east and west are discussed. This examination gives insight into just how many moving parts there were for a very long time, well into the mid to late 1800s, where issues and discussions between state, federal, and tribal authorities were mired in debate (55–59).

Ultimately, that separation of brothers and sisters in each of those Cherokee nations lasted until relatively recently, when the Cherokee Nation and the Eastern Band of Cherokee Indians met on ancestral council grounds at Red Clay, Tennessee, in 1984, 146 years after Removal. Wilma Mankiller, former chief of the Cherokee Nation, quietly cried at witnessing the eternal flame being brought from North Carolina by the young Cherokee runners: "As I stood there, I tried to imagine again the anger, frustration and passion my ancestors must have felt" (quoted in Sohn 2009).

Some today believe that many of those who left, particularly the Old Settlers (who migrated west by 1820), and some who sacrificed and faced many legal challenges to stay in North Carolina did so in an attempt to preserve their traditional way of life, traditional ceremonies, sacred places, and language. Hopefully, historians and cultural specialists within the Tribe will be able to add to what history is available today with greater insight into the creativity, forward thinking, and commitment to cultural preservation that was displayed during these chaotic and traumatic years of Removal and litigation.

Comparatively, there has been little written about the role Cherokee women played in keeping families and communities grounded during these times or their role during more traditional times. A woman's position in the home and council house was unlike anything Europeans had experienced. The eighteenth-century memoirist Henry Timberlake ([1765] 1948), commented: "These chiefs, or headmen, likewise compose the assemblies of the nation, into which the war women are admitted. The reader will not be a little surprised to find the story of Amazons not so great a fable as we imagined, many of the Indian women being as famous in war, as powerful in the council" (93).

For a broader and more enlightening discussion of how early English and Spanish explorers viewed Indigenous women, Louis Montrose's chapter in *New World Encounters* (1993), entitled "The Work of Gender in the Discourse of Discovery," provides readers with examples of Sir Walter Raleigh's "Western desire" to conquer the "feminine land" of the Guiana's Amazons (their warring women) and to support, reinforce, and promote the idea that the "Englishmen 'had many' of the Indian women in their power . . . [Raleigh] represents territorial conquest as the enforced defloration and possession of a female body" (183, 206). Raleigh used this discourse as a strategy in rationalizing his exploitation of the New World and in navigating his relationship with Queen Elizabeth.

Montrose goes on to make a point of Raleigh's violent and misogynistic mindset: "The object of this overdetermined desire encompasses identity and security, knowledge, wealth, and power. It seeks to know, master, and possess a feminized space—or, in the language of Raleigh's Virginia patent, 'to discover search fynde out and view . . . to have holde occupy and enjoye'; it is a desire that is most vividly realized as the prospect of deflowering a virgin" (206).

Not so surprising in a masculine-dominated world of exploration, other early travelers into Cherokee territory expressed deep concern and often hostility when witnessing women's prominence in early meetings and negotiations. Chief Indian agent Benjamin Hawkins, who served as a senator of North Carolina, wrote of his complete disdain for the power women held in matrilineal tribes. He provided an example of women among the Creek Nation—Hannah Hales "possesses the right of a Creek woman, and can throw away her husband whenever she chooses"—and continued that "he could not or would not accept their power in Creek social organization" (Henri 1986, 147). Historian Florette Henri (1986) says of Hawkins, "The matriarchal system so outraged his white-male sensibilities, and the thought that 'a whiteman by marrying an Indian woman . . . becomes a slave of her family' was so repugnant to him, that he issued an order forbidding, on pain of dismissal, any of his assistants to marry a Creek woman" (147).

As with Creeks, Cherokees were matrilineal and the women owned everything and made decisions regarding life and death in the council houses. They decided what would be planted and how much. They were highly regarded and played a major role in the life of every tribal member.

European contact and colonization changed everything, gender roles included. At a Timberlake memoirs symposium in 2006, historian and Cherokee studies scholar William Anderson spoke about these changes: "Paths to male bonding were disappearing by the 1700s. Dragging Canoe (Tsiyu Gan[a]sini, ᏥᏳ ᎦᎾᏏᏂ), a Chickamauga Cherokee warrior and leader well known for his efforts to preserve his culture and homeland, was trying to go by the old laws even though he was a young man. The Cherokee Lighthorse guard signaled decline of the clan system, and within forty years of Timberlake's visit, matrilineality was in decline." Speaking at the same symposium, Cherokee elder and language scholar Tom Belt agreed, pointing to the rapid changes of the 1700s: "We would have never gone against the wishes of the clan mothers. We had to have peace to afford more time to rebuild the culture." Some estimate that up to two-thirds of Cherokee populations died from smallpox epidemics before 1762. After the Anglo-Cherokee War in the early 1760s, General Rutherford's orchestrated moves on the eve of the revolution destroyed most of the Cherokee Middle and Valley Towns, along with their subsistence crops, leaving them to disease and starvation, not to mention lasting physical and emotional trauma. Tom continued, "The Kituwah way of life was super stressed. Timberlake was witnessing a process of surviving under duress with local wars, displacement, and the decline of matrilineality."

Even in the 1790s Cherokee women's councils mediated conflicts and treaties. In *Separate Peoples, One Land*, Cynthia Cumfer (2007) stresses how Cherokees incorporated clan and kinship models in their verbiage of treaties and negotiations with increasingly encroaching non-Natives:

> [Cherokee leader] Nan-ye-hi's assertion of a universal humanity rooted in a diplomatic motherhood was affirmed by five older members of the Women's Council, who addressed [General Nathan] Greene's conference on behalf of the women at the conclusion of the 1781 peace talks. They sought to bolster their authority by having a male chief, Scolacutta, accompany them. They

whispered their speech to him, which he delivered to the assembled audience. Unfortunately, only part of their remarkable address was preserved:

> We the women of the Cherokee nation now speak to you. We are
> mothers and have many sons, some of them warriors and be-
> loved men. We call you also our sons. We have a right to call you
> so, because you are the sons of mothers, and all descended from
> the same woman at first. We say you are our sons, because by
> women, you were brought forth into this world, nursed, suckled,
> and raised up to be men before you reached your present great-
> ness. Why should there be any difference amongst us? We live on
> the same land as you, and our people are mixed with white blood:
> one third of our [people are] mixed with white blood. (37–38)

Cumfer goes on to explain that "building on Nan-ye-hi's construction, these women imagined a diplomatic motherhood linked to Selu, the first woman and a powerful spiritual figure. They reminded Anglo men of the importance of women, a point that was critical because women's energy was needed to balance male forces" (38). This research is even more powerful in that the Cherokee women's council work would ultimately influence the diplomacy of human rights and international law.

By the early 1800s Cherokees were facing a very different and new world imposed on them by wars and colonizing efforts of those who came to exploit. Brett H. Riggs (1999) observes that "social and religious organizations had been crippled by wartime loss of essential personnel and the periodic jarring displacements of Cherokee settlements" (54). He explains, "While many Cherokees struggled to maintain a traditional lifestyle based on the fur trade and subsistence horticulture, they grew increasingly impoverished relative to their mid-Eighteenth Century prosperity. A deep sense of cultural disorientation, social dissolution and material poverty gripped the Cherokees at the end of the eighteenth century" (54).

What most historians do not accentuate in the Cherokees' evolution of acculturation (perhaps because these historians have in large part been men) is that Cherokee social stability and structure had been breached by the subjection of matrilineal society, which was transformed into a patriarchal mirror of the colonizers. An acknowledgment of matrilineality and a clan-based social organization survived the first five centuries of colonization, but what more about the roles and responsibilities of women was diminished or completely eradicated?

Anthropologist Raymond D. Fogelson (1977), who conducted research among the Cherokees from the 1950s into the twenty-first century, recognized historically the crucial role that Cherokee women played in activities relating to war. John Gulick (1960), drawing on Fogelson's ethnographic contributions, discusses the survival of the clan system as indicative of the shift in centrality of women in Cherokee society. Gulick notes that "the old town organization, in which there was a council organized by clan, was generally defunct long before the Removal, . . . the standard American family name system—patrilineal—has been used by all Eastern Cherokees since the middle of the nineteenth century, . . . [and] the non-Indian inheritance of many Eastern Cherokees has tended to weaken the clan system by removing people from possible clan membership" (65–66). Gulick goes on to cite several surveys on clan knowledge from the 1930s to the late 1950s reflecting a decrease in adherence to and knowledge of clan affiliations.

To know who you are, an identity that could only originate from your biological mother, sets the stage for all other activity and responsibility in Cherokee society. The roles and positions of women were attacked from the very beginning of contact with Europeans, who stripped matrilineally based societies of their stability, structure, and core identity. As Native psychologist Eduardo Duran (2004) has explained, the patrilineal, male-centered spirit of the Western world came to the female-centered societies of the western hemisphere to dominate, subjugate, and rape the culture and land. It is no accident that the land, Mother Earth, and environmental issues are synonymous with women.

In the chapter "Sacred Feminine in Cherokee Culture," Jenny James (2009) notes that "the matriarchal structures of consciousness present in Cherokee texts (whether myth or medical formulas) encompass feminine patterns of cultural reconstruction and restoration, and delineate multiple levels of sacred feminine meaning, which are present in the psyche. Fire, Corn, Sun, and Stars are several of the cosmological referents of the Great Mother archetype in Cherokee culture, and these figures and their root metaphors encrypt the nature of feminine sensibility for Cherokee spiritual transformation." She asks, "Without these structures of the sacred feminine, how can one access religious meaning in a matriarchal culture such as Cherokee culture?" (117).

In looking at leadership in the EBCI community today, we find many examples of women holding important positions of authority in areas of law, health, and education. But there is continued need for women to recognize their heritage and reclaim their rightful place in the civil and cultural structures of Kituwah communities, to facilitate healing families and eradicate violence against women, which is a national and urgent issue in Indian country.

Women of Kituwah today have much to be proud of in this heritage. It has been said at community meetings with elders that it will only be possible to heal the serious social ills of Cherokee communities through their women.

Women's reclaiming of positions of power and respect can help eradicate issues of violence against women and children, and ultimately address the urgent environmental issues that we face locally and globally as well. If one accepts the crucial position of women in Kituwah or Cherokee society historically and culturally, how then can one argue with those elders speaking about the critical need for women to restore healing in today's communities?

Hopefully more Cherokee and Indigenous women will contribute to the dialogue about place, identity, responsibility, and healing. They are, and always have been, the glue that keeps families together and the fearless activists that participated in the challenges colonization brought to Native communities.

Chapter Three

◇◇◇◇◇◇◇◇◇◇◇◇◇◇◇◇◇◇◇◇◇◇◇◇◇◇◇◇

WHEN THE LAND IS SICK, WE ARE SICK

Metaphysics of Indigenous Epistemologies

> Even our language reflects we are problem solvers.
> The science of how we live and how we relate to
> everything around us is protected in our language.
> Our language is more than just a code for English.
>
> THOMAS N. BELT

This book is not about how an anthropologist views or speaks for Indigenous peoples; it is about how Appalachian people and Indigenous people find common ground with the importance of place and identity. It is about how Indigenous peoples are speaking for all of us whose culture and heritage are directly attached to a place, a location, a geographic space. This homeland houses the natural diversity and ways of life and living that generations of people adapted to and have built a culture around. With that come the ways of knowing—the epistemologies—that provide us with guidance and understanding of how to live in the local world around us.

The Cherokee people have lived in one of the most biologically diverse ecosystems in the world long enough to have observed, field-tested, and inventoried thousands of flora and fauna, cosmological movements, climate change, and geological phenomena. By the time Europeans descended on them, they had highly developed agrarian methods and seed hybridization techniques that provided them with a wide variety of corn, beans, and squash, among many other domesticated plants. Simply put, Indigenous people had knowledge of genetics that was time tried over the long term and had, as a result, seeds and seed stock that were adaptable to place (Federoff 2003). Their botanical knowledge rivaled, if not surpassed, that of Western science at that time. Certainly they had more biodiversity with which to work. EBCI member Kevin Welch, founder and director of the Center for Cherokee Plants, explains: "As a people, we Cherokee have forgotten a large amount of our woodland knowledge, perhaps as much as 85–90 percent of our traditional uses for wild plants. The mountains of Southern Appalachia have a huge biodiversity and Cherokee people have had several thousand years to learn to use this resource. At one time, it would have been commonly known when, where and what plants and animals might be found during certain times of the year. Having this knowledge of available resources makes the difference between just living and living well!" (quoted in Veteto et al. 2011, 18).

The idea that the first inhabitants of the western hemisphere were unintelligent, primitive, or savage has been the one of the biggest lies of Western religion and education. Only in recent decades have texts been introduced to Western academies that contradict this notion by providing evidence to the contrary (as though "evidence" was necessary). We were taught that Indigenous peoples were "primitive," insinuating that they lacked curiosity, ingenuity, and intellectualism, a strategy to dehumanize and subjugate. Gregory Cajete in his chapter "Philosophy of Native Science" (2004) shows us just the opposite:

> Native science is a broad term that can include metaphysics and philosophy, art and architecture, practical technologies, and agriculture, as well as ritual and ceremony practiced by Indigenous peoples past and present. More specifically, Native science encompasses such areas as astronomy, farming, plant domestication, plant medicine, animal husbandry, hunting, fishing, metallurgy, geology—studies related to plants, animals, and natural phenomena, yet may extend to include spirituality, community, creativity, and technologies which sustain environments and support essential aspects of human life. It may even include exploration of such questions as the nature of language, thought, and perception, the movement of time and space, the nature of human knowing and feeling. . . . It has given rise to the diversity of human technologies, even to the advent of modern mechanistic science. (47)

We know that Indigenous knowledge has perpetuated an understanding of how we, as organic entities, are related or connected to all other natural things, and through modern physicists, we accept a modern, Western science to tell us that this is a valid paradigm. Vine Deloria Jr. (1979) wrote, "Our task is to discern from the continuous introduction of new elements of knowledge and experience a coherent interpretation of the scheme of things. Traditionally, Western people have called an inquiry of this kind *metaphysics*, and its task has been to discover the structure and meaning of what was real. The word itself has become somewhat frightening to Western peoples because of their inclination to make metaphysical conclusions an absolute canon of faith, thus imposing abstract principles on their practical understandings of the world around them." He goes on to discuss how Western peoples have discouraged the synthesis of "respective fields of knowledge into a coherent whole" (11).

Among Europeans this antisynthetic drive has been historically understood as the struggle between science and religion. However, Native thought dissolves this distinction. Dawn Martin-Hill (2008), a First Nations scholar, writes of Indigenous knowledge and power: "The cultural diversity of Indigenous peoples is addressed through the recognition that Indigenous knowledge is attached to the language, landscapes, and cultures from which it emerges" (8). It moves beyond the Western hierarchical system of knowledge, and it moves beyond just attachment to the land. She refers to Indigenous scholars Marie Battiste and James Henderson's explanation that "Indigenous peoples regard all products of the human mind and heart as interrelated with Indigenous knowledge. They assert that all knowledge flows from the same source: the relationships between a global flux that needs to be renewed; the people's kinship with other creatures who share the land; and the people's kinship with the spirit world." Martin-Hill summarizes that "the validity of Indigenous knowledge is noted in Indigenous universal natural law, which posits that knowledge is spiritually based and ecologically derived" (10).

For us as Westerners to broaden our understanding of how we are connected to all things, and how those connections can make us healthier and more whole, we can best turn to the epistemologies and ways of doing conveyed through Indigenous language and practices. Deloria knew this as well. He begins in his book *Metaphysics of Modern Existence* (1979), "The fundamental factor that keeps Indians and non-Indians from communicating is that they are speaking about two entirely different perceptions of the world" (vii). His elaboration of this is fundamental in how we come to know Native science and how it can make for realistic application in health care and environmental conservation, two fields that many in the Western academy also see as distantly related at best.

Deloria explains, "Growing up on a reservation makes one acutely aware of the mysteries of the universe. Medicine men practicing their ancient ceremonies perform feats that amaze and puzzle the rational mind. The sense of contentment enjoyed by older Indians in the face of a lifetime's experience of betrayal, humiliation, and paternalism stuns the astute observer. It often appears that Indians are immune to the values which foreign institutions have forced them to confront. Their minds remain fixed on other realities." He continues, "In a white man's world, knowledge is a matter of memorizing theories, dates, lists of kings and presidents, the table of chemical elements, and many other things not encountered in the course of a day's work. Knowledge seems to be divorced from experience. Even religion is a process of memorizing creeds, catechisms, doctrines, and dogmas—general principles that never seem to catch the essence of human existence. No matter how well educated an Indian may become, he or she also suspects that Western culture is not an adequate representation of reality . . . the trick is somehow to relate what one feels with what one is taught to think" (vii).

As an anthropologist for almost three decades working in Native communities with Native people of varying backgrounds and beliefs, I have heard for many years statements like "we are relatives of all that live around us, including the stars in the universe." For a social scientist, this simple statement is layered with complex, yet clear meaning: Native peoples have known for thousands of years that we are all made up of the same "stuff." We are not only *in* nature, but *of* nature. My lack of understanding as an academic was challenged by my understanding as an Appalachian person who had spent much time with family outside, with nature. My mother would often remark that we are part of a magnificent and wonderous place, if we only took time to be a part of it and understand it. So, I was more apt to listen to elders in ceremony who spoke about our relationship with the world around us. My problem was making it fit with my ego of academic professionalism. As Deloria (1979) put it: "Western people don't have a problem—they don't seem concerned with the ultimate truth of what they are taught—Knowledge is correlated with a higher status employment. . . . Indian customs and beliefs were regarded as primitive, superstitions, and unworthy of serious attention. . . . So the question of the validity of knowledge contained in Indian traditions was eliminated before any discussions of reality began" (viii).

In 2010 at Western Carolina University we started a symposium called Rooted in the Mountains: Valuing Our Common Ground. This conference is intended to integrate traditional knowledge with health and environmental issues. We bring locals, both Native and non-Native Appalachian people, together with Western-trained scientists to discuss topics that affect all our lives. It is our hope and belief that these discussions exemplify the common ground we share and value the knowledge that comes from many different perspectives. We also think it is important that these discussions occur at a local university where, historically, these views, languages, and people have not been well understood or valued.

In 2011, Western Carolina University and the Center for Native Health hosted the first Native Science Dialogues on the East Coast. Nine Native scientists came from almost as many tribes to discuss the application of their epistemologies and language to the mission of the ongoing discussions at our

Rooted in the Mountains meetings. David Begay, a Diné elder, commented about Indian students in the academy:

> American Indian students go to universities alone. No one understands them. They go through and get their degrees but can't apply them at home. Universities don't serve everybody or all of an individual—only a piece of their needs. You have to create a model of interdisciplinary work. The world of interrelationship means things don't happen on their own. Native people have a hard time thinking in a separated world. You must be able to process how the world is interconnected. English compartmentalizes stuff. It puts humans in the middle, whereas most Native languages don't. The center of the language is nature, not man. Life must come first. The law of entropy means the land will restore itself. Go and ask elders regarding a process to manage renewal, and they will say look at nature with the daily, weekly, monthly, seasonal processes—they are all in nature.

Speaking at the Dialogues, Leroy Little Bear, a Blackfoot elder and Indigenous physicist, asked how we respond to the notion that "when the land is sick, I am sick, and when I am sick, the land is sick." Begay responded: "In Navajo, the word for land is *shike'yah*, which means the connection to earth under the moccasins. My mother is *shima'*, which means like a mother and infant relationship. *Shi-*, the root in each word, links the meanings together. This land is our mother earth, not just land or dirt, but the earth that has a bond with us like a mother does with her infant child. They are inseparable."

Words and language are critically important in understanding Indigenous worldviews as is exemplified by the discussions of Tom and others in this book. As F. David Peat (2002) found in his work with Blackfoot and other tribal elders and speakers, "within Indigenous science, thoughts are inseparable from language. The language that is spoken is not simply a medium, or a vehicle for communication, rather it is a living thing, an actual physical power within the universe. The vibrations of its words are energies that act within the transforming processes we call reality. Moreover, each language is a link with the particular landscape in which a people live" (224).

Speaking at the 2011 Dialogues, Jim Rock, a Dakota Native scientist and principal investigator on the final NASA space shuttle mission (also in 2011), said that the longest distance is often between the heart and mind. He said, "When we breathe in air, we are where space and earth meet. The breath goes out to the trees. We're all in space, not welcoming, but dark and cold—the breath, however, unites us all. Our heart beats and keeps us warm. Of course we're all connected, all just to love each other as we love Mother Earth."

In a 2011 meeting regarding Indigenous land rights held at Wake Forest

University, Greg Johnson from the University of Colorado spoke about his work among Native Hawaiians and relayed how they talk about their land. He said that their talk usually fell in one of six categories of the sacred: (1) places unto themselves—sites of power or "vectors of energy" (e.g., mountaintops and some types of springs); (2) ceremonial sites—places both ancient and contemporary that were historically important and used for life-cycle rituals; (3) sites of violence—places of personal pilgrimage, dance, meditation, and historical travel; (4) subsistence sites—seen as problematic by colonizers, places that were host to traditional agricultural practices and products that were culturally identified and are central to mythology and belief (he noted that sacred agricultural rituals are now rare but should have heightened significance for tribes); (5) defiled places—sites that have been abused, defiled, and exploited and now require spiritual/religious care from those who understand their cosmological and cultural association with land; and (6) burial sites—places where a direct connection to the land is made, sometimes also representing ongoing life, energy activity, and protection for ancestors.

In terms of our connectedness to land, and in our case in Southern Appalachia, we as mountain people identify with the land. We are the people of Appalachia. I've heard that the mountains protect us, they nurture us, they identify who we are, and they help heal us. Appalachian writer Wendell Berry (1995) writes of health and wellness. He says, "If you are going to deal with the issue of health in the modern world, you are going to have to deal with much absurdity. . . . The modern medical industry faithfully imitates disease in the way that it isolates us and parcels us out. If, for example, intense and persistent pain causes you to pay attention only to your stomach, then you must leave home, community, and family and go to a sometimes distant clinic or hospital, where you will be cared for by a specialist who will pay attention only to your stomach. . . . I believe that health is wholeness. For many years I have turned again and again to the work of English agriculturist Sir Albert Howard, who said, in *The Soil and Health*, that 'the whole problem of health in soil, plant, animal, and man [is] one great subject'" (88–90). Berry continues, "I believe that the community—in the fullest sense: a place and all its creatures—is the smallest unit of health and that to speak of the health of an isolated individual is a contradiction in terms" (90).

Growing up in Appalachia, I understood that there was a deep and important connection between people and the natural world. I was in awe of the diversity around us, whether it be plants, animals, water, rocks, or wind that was always welcomed. Spending time in the forests made me keenly aware of how dependent we are on everything around us. Because of my mother's expertise in use of medicinal plants, I also knew that most ailments took more than one plant to help, and that for every ailment, there was a cure in those mountains.

Another example comes from the work of Tommie Bass, an herbalist from northern Alabama. After my mother got to the place where she could no longer make the medicines she wanted, I was pleased to find the work and medicines of Mr. Bass. I found one of his skin creams being sold at a store in Cherokee, and it contained the same ingredients that my mom used to use. My mother and maternal uncle, both of whom suffered from recurrent skin cancers, used this cream or salve with great success.

When "Cherokee medicine" is spoken of, most people think of going into the mountains and gathering a plant to be used for healing a specific ailment. It is much more complicated and sophisticated than that. One must consider a larger contextual environment that is critical in Cherokee medicinal practices. This is why so much caution is associated with protecting "sacred formulas." It is more to protect those who would use the formulas. The adage "a little knowledge is a dangerous thing" comes to mind. It has been said that there are protocols for plant usage and other medicinal usages to protect the person who is using the medicine. Without knowing the full context of where, when, and why particular medicines are used, you can do more harm than good. It takes years of learning, watching, listening, and understanding the Cherokee language to appropriately administer the full potential of Cherokee medicine.

Some might want to seek out a sacred text and have it translated to extract information about the medicinal use of a plant or plants. Without knowledge of the Cherokee language and the meaning that accompanies the process of application, the information about directional use, and all of the other nuances that are embedded in the language, you are not using Cherokee medicine. This is a science that has come from millennia of measurement, observation, and trial and error. Even the act of going to a river, stream, mountainside, or valley and collecting a plant is incomplete without knowledge of a broader linguistic context. How would one know which plant within a group of plants is the right one to collect? How would one know what time of day or season is the most appropriate for plant collection? How would one know what should be said during plant collection and transportation? How would one know exactly what combination and amount of plants should be used for specific ailments or specific patients? These factors are all a part of the science.

Eduardo Duran, a Native psychologist and pioneer of the "soul wound" model, prominent in counseling Native populations, addressed a group of Cherokee health providers and other clinicians in 2010. He spoke of the responsibility of clinicians to integrate Native "ways of doing and thinking" in their service to Cherokee people. The Western-trained health provider is taught to externally treat a patient, to treat a problem and not a whole person, to rely on medication, pills, and liquids that quickly take effect and treat illness.

Duran's perspective was that the money-based, multinational pharmaceutical corporations embrace a spirit that is counterproductive to the healing process. Indigenous processes of healing operate from the inside out. It isn't that some medications are ineffective. We know that an overwhelming majority of pharmaceuticals are derivatives of plants. However, along with the escalating pharmaceutical costs, issues of addiction, and side effects associated with prescription pill use comes what many Native traditionalists refer to as a negative spirit of production and exploitation. The inference from many elders like Duran is that we rape the land and force commercial growth of life-giving plants to be exploited by corporations. We forget the healing spirit and protocols that respect the earth, plants, water, and other natural resources, which provide us with healing properties.

So as we reflect on our connection with the earth and all that is on it, we can easily find examples of how toxic dumps, coal mining, and polluted water make people sick. There are serious consequences for rural people who witness the destruction of their land. My mother, who was rather stoic and did not show expression of pain or sorrow often, would reflexively wince and even shed tears at mountainsides that were scarred from "development" or unfinished dozing. It was as if someone had cut or scarred her, an empathetic response that showed her distress over what she considered mistreatment of the mountains.

Glenn Albrecht (2010) writes that depression, sadness, and consuming distress are "human response[s] to the lived experience of an emerging negative relationship to a home environment" (230). Love for our land and strong identity with place are said to be part of an organic interconnection linking humans and their environment. There are many languages that categorize the extreme unbalance people feel when their physical world changes rapidly, but English is not one of them. The Inuit, Hopi, and even Portuguese have language to express the distress of "unwelcomed disturbance to their home environments" (Albrecht 2010, 217). Albrecht coins the terms "psychoterratic" and "somaterratic" to characterize the relationship between health and environment: loss of one's home environment can cause mental and physical illness, while a "positive relationship to a loved home environment delivers the benefits of a strong endemic sense of place and enhanced well-being" (217–18).

The triumphs of the Wampanoag of Massachusetts at rebirthing their language are brilliantly captured in a film by Anne Makepeace entitled *We Still*

Live Here (2010). In it, tribal member Jesse Little Doe Baird speaks of how in their language, "for the Wampanoag people to lose one's land, to lose the rights for use of our land is to literally fall off your feet—to have no ground under you. The word *matake'* means 'my land is not separate from my body, and my land is attached to my feet, whatever I do.'" She also points out in a language lesson that the nouns for stars and moon are animate because they move, whereas the sun is inanimate. She said, "the Wampanoag people knew the sun didn't move, but the moon did. Europeans just figured that out a few hundred years ago."

I have heard on many occasions Hopi, Navajo, Kiowa, Cherokee, and other tribal elders speak of having to learn to get back to who they are, knowing their place in the world and universe. They have talked about the children being sent off to boarding school and taught to lose their language and awareness of relationships. Through traditional ceremony and seasonal ritual their place in the universe was remembered. One Hopi elder said in the 2011 land rights meeting, "It's hard to talk about who we are as Indian people using English language. Western culture even ten years ago didn't recognize our knowledge. Now it is time to bring it into Western culture. The 'American Dream' is about wealth, real estate, and individuality, but that way of thinking has brought about loss, pain, isolation, and separation. We must teach about how we think in terms of seven generations, and we meditate to make connections with the heart of people. Ingratitude takes away from meditation and our awareness of connection to everything around us. We are taught [in Western society] to honor individualism instead of all of our relations." A colleague reminded me that the English term "real estate" implies transaction, ownership: "ownership" of property makes it *real* to English speakers. It implies privatization, in stark contrast to the worldview of Wampanoag and other Native peoples.

The ancient knowledge of connection to all else around us is being understood through the work of Native scientists and physicists. Today's technology reinforces the teachings of Indigenous people that we are all related as we are all made of the same matter. We are swimming in a constantly moving sea of energy that is influenced by our behaviors, and some will say even our thoughts. Several years ago, I listened to an interview on National Public Radio with Jill Bolte Taylor, a neuroanatomist and national spokesperson for the Harvard Brain Tissue Resource Center (and one of *Time* magazine's Hundred Most Influential People in the World for 2008). In the 2008 interview, she spoke of her book *My Stroke of Insight* (2009) and discussed the notion that energy is emitted in all things around us and that the brain is able to tap into and process this activity at some level. She writes: "As information processing machines, our ability to process data about the external world begins at the level of sensory perception. Although most of us are rarely aware of it, our sensory receptors are designed to detect information at the energy level. Because everything around us—the air we breathe, even the materials we use to build with—are composed of spinning and vibrating atomic particles, you and I are literally swimming in a turbulent sea of electromagnetic fields. We are part of it. We are enveloped within it, and through our sensory apparatus we experience what is" (18). What came to my mind was the universal Indigenous paradigm, "we are all connected." It is being proven by sciences from neuroanatomy to metaphysics. We aren't just all connected to one another; we are connected to every other living thing on this planet.

Even if we may not be conscious of our relationship to the natural world, some Indigenous traditions reflect that it is aware of us. For example, in Cherokee and Mohawk stories, it is understood that plants are here to help us. As Mohawk elder Katsi Cook (2018) said, "plants are the only living things that will come all the way to your door to try to help you if you let them. Medicine is out there to help us. We have that for our disposal if we know how to do that, if we understand it, and we know how to use it. If we don't know, it's best not to mess with it." But recognizing we are part of that natural world and understanding that we have a relationship to maintain is a critical part of being healthy and thereby keeping the world healthy. If we can begin to think more like our Indigenous brothers and sisters, we might have a chance of ecological and health renewal and a more effective and useful understanding of obtaining true health and wellness.

Chapter Four

THE LAND KEEPS OUR HISTORY
AND IDENTITY

Cherokee and Appalachian Cosmography

> Being here is a gift. We are guests. It was here before
> we came. We weren't even first! It was the plants
> and the animals and later we came. It was all here
> before we came, and it will be here after we leave.
> Our obligation is to take care of it and respect it.
>
> THOMAS N. BELT

Native peoples are the most intelligent, generous, kind, and interesting people I've had the honor to know. It has been the most rewarding experience to get to know these individuals and their homelands. I will forever remember those with whom I've worked, dined, played, and had ceremony. So much was shared as we traveled through their lands, in and by rivers and streams, watching animals and walking through forests, each venture reinforcing that we are all connected and we are all relatives. Whether we were in the desert, near the ocean, in the mountains, or on the plains, where we saw stars in the sky and they would talk of history and express their intellect, they understood their place in the universe. Or, as T. J. Holland (EBCI) says, it is "understanding our traditional landscape as our *cosmography*."

They would talk of their relations to all that we could see and hear and to what they could not see or hear, way ahead of their Western counterparts, who were several thousand years behind in physics. Places where we had watched children grow, people marry, folks be buried, where they—a people whose humor, resilience, and adaptation are truly wonders—had seen challenges and worked diligently to overcome them, all of these places and spaces had deep and abiding meaning and anchored them.

In 2010 Silas House, award-winning Appalachian writer, was keynote speaker at Western Carolina University's first Rooted in the Mountains Symposium. In that year, Silas spoke of "thin places" for mountain people, places where this world and the spirit world meet. He said, "I did not know a time when the mountain was not there, a wall and a guard, a protector and an obstacle, a presence larger than anything else, an entity that dictated where water flowed, where people put their homes and trailers and churches, where the roads were able to cut through. The boss. The mountain was our past and our present, our family and our future, our whole identity as a way of life." Silas went on to speak of those times when someone's passing or other trauma was experienced and his family would go up on the mountain to a place where this world and the spirit world were so close one could feel the presence of the divine. These were healing places. Places where one's soul could be refreshed and peace was a veil that washed over them. Those places existed for many in Appalachia, Native and non-Native alike. They may not have been the same places, but they were there.

In the Rooted symposiums, we have heard from others who have spoken about the importance of these sacred places, for us as Appalachian people and for the Kituwah or Cherokee, the first inhabitants of these mountains. In 2018 for the annual Appalachian Studies Association conference, I organized a panel where Appalachian writers and Cherokee community members spoke of this topic again. The meeting provided a forum for discussion of these places and the ways they sustain us, heal us, and provide a core identity for those of us who claim cultural heritage of being Appalachian.

In Ireland and Scotland, "thin places" are nationally identified and protected. Novels have been written about them, pilgrimages have been organized around them, and families' oral histories keep their locations as a refuge for difficult times. Because my grandfather's land was sold when I was very young and my parents had no landholdings, my mother relegated her visits to those thin places to land that was accessible, often land of distant cousins or national park land. Later as more and more private land that she had known well as a child was sold and fenced off, accessibility to those places was prohibitive. She encouraged me to find places that were powerful and comforting, that allowed me to feel close to the sacred. In reality they aren't hard to find. But once you have found them, you must be respectful and recognize their importance. There are those places that my mom and I shared and other places that I later learned had been embraced and protected by the first inhabitants of this land. These are those places and features of our surroundings that demand us to acknowledge their presence, their power, and their identity in helping us be resilient and connected.

Presenting in a 2019 international conference on mountains, Appalachian author Pamela Y. Duncan said, "There are still those for whom place is a sacred repository of history, culture, and identity. Even after the loss of a home place, the land itself remains, peopled by the ghosts of lives lived there. They recognized creation as sacred and behaved in ways that honored that sacredness."

For mountain people thin places can be as simple as a rock on the mountain or a mossy place by a creek or river. For Kituwahs who have lived here for millennia, there may be a physical mark on a rock or land feature that indicates its long identification as a place of communication or direction or ritual. There may be markings along a river that reflect activity of Uktena (ᎤᎦᏔᎾ), a large horned serpent that resided in the water of Kituwah country, a place where a powerful Tsanusi (ᏣᏄᏏ) or leech lived, a mound such as Nikwasi (ᏂᏆᏏ), which connected Kituwahs with the stars in the heavens, or Judaculla Rock (ᎤᏣᏍᏗ ᏚᏩᎣᏫ), where a giant left his mark as a reminder of places where people would be taught.

Judaculla Rock (figure 4.1) is an important place in Cherokee cosmography in that it marks the site where the giant Tsul'kala (ᏚᏩᎣᏫ, Judaculla) landed when he jumped from the "Devil's Courthouse," a mountain just north of Caney Fork in Jackson County. Judaculla was a teacher and warrior. Judaculla Rock is the largest petroglyph in the eastern United States. Its lines and markings are part of the teachings of the Kituwah people. The mark of the six-fingered hand of Judaculla himself connects this significant place with several other petroglyphs that run through the ancient Cherokee territory of western North Carolina. Tom has explained to visitors here that Cullowhee, about three miles away and the home of Western Carolina University, is the namesake of Judaculla; "Cullowhee" means "Judaculla's place."

Judaculla's place, the whole valley in which the university sits, has historically been a place of teaching and learning. Unfortunately, in the 1950s as the need for expansion came, a large mound was torn down, reflective of a lingering colonial mindset and disregard for this important ancient place. More recently a site, *tali tsisgwayahi* (ᏔᎵ ᏥᏍᏆᏯᎯ, Two Sparrows Town), was discovered as room was made to expand the campus for much-needed space. Fortunately, those archaeologists and Cherokee studies faculty at the university came together to carefully preserve the site and partner with the Eastern Band of Cherokee Indians to use this information to teach about Kituwah people for generations to come. This may be one of the oldest Cherokee sites ever found (for photos, see WCU, n.d.). Tom emphasizes how these places teach him about his heritage and confirm his identity as a Cherokee person and this land as his homeland.

Non-Natives might visit these places as tourists, admiring the identification of Kituwahs' long history and culture. But we should keep in mind these

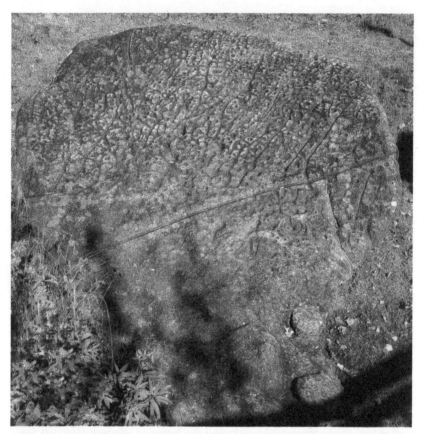

Figure 4.1. Judaculla Rock, Jackson County, North Carolina. Courtesy of Rosemary Peek.

are sacred places that can teach everyone about how to live by understanding their stories and language. These are places where we can all find peace by being resolute in their protection for perpetuity. As Tom has said often, part of being sacred means it has meaning and purpose for all.

Unfortunately, many Kituwah youth don't recognize the importance of these places, not only for confirming one's identity, but for providing solace and healing. We tend to limit ourselves to a short radius, only that county or acreage we are most familiar with, but Cherokee youth can be proud that the history and legacy of their ancestors extends across hundreds of miles of territory, crossing counties and states. In the past they understood their environment, were masters of environmental stewardship, and had untold numbers of sites for ceremony and prayer. Their homeland for so many thousands of years fed them and provided them with the resources they needed to build towns, homes, and transport far past their own territory. Cherokee youth can be proud of a strong, rich, and abundant heritage in which a unique language was created to characterize and explain a way of life that still exists and brings honor to this place and its accompanying worldview. English does not and cannot do that. The connected systems of life in the soil, plants, sky, valleys, rivers, and mountains have laws and rules of behavior and interaction that elders consider natural laws. These laws are in place to ensure good health and well-being.

In talking with a young Cherokee student who was interested in how place heals, Tom Belt mentioned the power the mountains hold in allowing us to climb them, look out and around and see the landscape of valleys and ridges in the distance, and see that we are very small in contrast—at the same time as we see that we are a real part of this place and it is a part of us. That connectedness brings wholeness and comfort for mountain people. He says, "It becomes a part of you and in doing so gives you a sense of confidence and comfort. It will always be here—it will go on. Knowing your connectedness is like a mechanism for how life works, we aren't in charge of it for it is greater than us; understanding it doesn't mean manipulating it."

It takes sometimes many years of walking the mountains to gain a sufficient familiarity, not only with place, but with the plants, birds, insects, and other animals that exist there, to know that as the seasons change, plants avail themselves, making themselves visible, ready for appreciation and use when needed. They are friends, they are food, and they are medicine. I remember my mother taking me with her on her frequent walks and giving me instructions to sit on a rock near a stream or creek and to "be still." When she returned, she would ask me: What did you hear? What did you see? She, like many who spent time in the forests, learned to appreciate different seasons, different latitudes, different times of the day to teach us about life going on all the time whether we were present or not. It allowed me to appreciate the sounds and smells and sights of a world that had its own pace. It gave me peace and comfort to know I was part of something so beautiful and interconnected. I will always be appreciative of that gift that she gave to me. It is priceless for keeping me sane, and also critically relevant in our troubled societies. The gift of nature as a therapeutic practice is invaluable.

A direct and immediate opportunity for the application of traditional knowledge is the development of mental health treatment and counseling approaches for Native populations. Native psychologists such as Eduardo Duran and Joseph P. Gone have been writing and speaking about this for several years, encouraging the development of unique tribal models that incorporate the perspectives and language of tribal elders and speakers, bringing ancient philosophies and ways of knowing to contemporary mental health issues.

Factors complicating the development of these more specific, traditional, tribal models include the Christianization of tribal people and varying degrees of assimilation and acculturation. The more than 50 percent of tribal people whose families were part of the federal relocation program in the 1950s, and who have become so-called urban Indians, may also not have access to tribally specific models or tribal speakers to assist in developing more culturally appropriate models of treatment or counseling, let alone have access to ancient, sacred sites of ceremonial healing.

Therefore, the task at hand is to determine how the development of these approaches can meet the needs of such varied and richly unique populations and still honor tribal culture and identity and be easily relatable to Native people.

In working with Cherokee elders and speakers on how to approach serious mental health issues for their people, bilingual speakers have facilitated the translation and retranslation from English to Cherokee and back to English of various basic mental health and wellness concepts such as depression or imbalance. In these rich and enlightening discussions, ancient philosophies and beliefs that anchor one's perceptions of self in the larger world have become apparent and are critical in finding stasis and wholeness in one's life.

These discussions reflect the traditional knowledge of the Kituwah people of North Carolina, but of course similar discussions could be taking place in Native-speaking communities all over. In the words of tribal cultural resources officer T. J. Holland, cosmography *is* traditional knowledge. It is the connection of Indigenous peoples to place and history and the cultural knowledge that has been passed down about meaning and importance of place.

What is critical for this and future generations of Kituwah people, is the real application of this type of knowledge, embedded in language, to the understanding of who they are, what they've been, how they have known their place in the world, and how this brings balance and healing. Many elders feel the only way to do this is to go back to an ancient way of thinking and knowing, one that aligns people with their home and their place in this world.

Tom Belt says, "It is language that teaches us that we are part of the land and the sky, connected to the natural world in both a cognitive and spiritual way." Even the name of the people who have occupied the southern Appalachians for more than twelve thousand years reflects their birthplace in how they identify themselves. Kituwah means we are of this place, we are of the earth, given to us by Creator. It also means a place called Kituwah, which is located just outside of Cherokee, North Carolina. Cherokee was a trade name given by outsiders. Tom continues, "Kituwah tells us who we are, where we are from, and who we will always be. It tells us that we are not just *from* this place, but *of* it."

This notion of place and identity is essential, a core element of healing. Those who have suffered from mental health problems, depression, addiction, and trauma must, in the words of one elder, "come home." Healing can only come from coming home and becoming very clear about who you are as a Kituwah. On the surface, this direction of discussion may seem inappropriate or ancillary to a mental health professional or social worker who is dealing with someone who is Native. However, as has been discussed among speakers, "if you are 'obsessing' [e.g., addicted, neurotic] you are taking yourself away from reality. A 'normal path or journey' isn't possible because you cannot be in this world understanding realistically what you must do to continue on your journey if you are constantly thinking of yourself or what or who you are obsessing about." Connecting with place grounds you to reality.

When Tom came back to North Carolina and found the place Kituwah, that place that his grandmother had described to him, he said, "Finding this place, this valley, this field, became who I was. I became connected to it immediately. Not just through stories or what I had read, but it affirmed to me the reality of my connection and identified who I am. It's not ownership—not the European idea of 'this is mine'—but this is my origin; I am looking at my mother." It made him complete. He continued, "It is like no other place." The connection made him whole.

Likewise, the notion of "depression" is translated *esga* (ᏕᏍᎦ, back toward you) *uyelvha* (ᎤᏰᎵᏆ, they are thinking that way), or, translated back into English, "all of their thoughts are directed back toward themselves." According to Cherokee elders, "You are supposed to look forward, as Creator put your eyes in front of your face." They also included, "This is why we didn't fear passage. We are curious people, always looking forward to more of life. We didn't focus on self because if we looked on the self constantly we die, we consume self by not looking outward. Likewise, the concepts of being angry, *unalv* (ᎤᎾᎳ), and being offended, *gvyuga* (ᎡᎪᏍ, they are offended), come from the root word for disease, *vyuga* (ᎢᎪᏍ)." In the Cherokee story of the emergence of disease, during the time when plants and animals could talk and the human latecomers could understand them, humans "offended" the animals by overkilling and exploiting them, so the animals gave them *vyuga*, disease. Plants then told the humans that they would help them by providing the medicine they needed to combat disease and provide balance (Mooney [1891–1900] 1982, 250). The elders continued, noting that language teaches us to connect with the land and environment in both a cognitive and a spiritual way.

As mental health concepts are discussed by Native-speaking elders, they share a linguistically preserved knowledge of human behavior, a science of critical elements of relationships, and an understanding through thousands of years of adaptation of what they see as "natural laws" that guide what they feel are truths that have been systematically observed, tested, and retested, that have proven critical in their resiliency as a people. Central here is their understanding of "the way" or "the road" that governs all, translated from the Cherokee *duyuk'dv'i*. One elder said, "All health-care providers must be on the same page, must be oriented to our cultural concepts and a health curricula which encompasses all that has to do with *duyuk'dv'i*, our concept of life, of wellness. To make this work, we must find people who will understand its importance and comply with these cultural laws. They must make a commitment to culture." *Duyuk'dv'i* is also understood as life energy. We are all moving forward, moving not necessarily in a straight line, but moving in a decided circle that is complete and includes our life cycle. We are in a steady flow and live as we are "supposed to" without stopping, but looking onward, forward, outward, being concerned for others, for the world around us. Things may happen in our life that make us step off the path, but we do what we need to do in order to continue to move forward and see *tohi* (health, wellness) and move back on the white path or right path. This is understood by Kituwahs as a natural and universal law.

Cherokees speak of the white path or narrow road, which is the color of the south, associated with light and warmth. This path is the anchor that never dies or goes away. In today's society, people speak of others who are their anchor, but sometimes, when these people die, it leaves those who have relied on them in distress or lost. A path, or way of life does not; rather, it is what identifies you as who you are. This path is lined with happiness and safety, and all other species, flora and fauna, follow it as well. One elder commented, "Was a time when there were no paupers or orphans in our Nation. Kinship and identity and the Kituwah way of life made sure you were never alone." He continued, "It is the language of our people that provides that connection, beliefs, and the way—it is the anchor."

One also must first understand that these elders aren't speaking of these laws as religious or "Christian." These are ancient ways of knowing that circumvent such categories and are more aptly understood by elders as "an old way of knowing," a science built on thousands of years of observation, reflection, and coding. An elder explained by saying, "This old way of knowing is one that is centered by relationships we have as human beings with nature around us in the biological world and to land, to the sky, to place, and the importance that comes from these connections and relationships that grounds us and centers us and teaches us how to be *tohi* [well]. The importance of who we are and our connection with place, how we live with others, including nonhuman beings, and how long we have had these relations is at the core of wellness. It is tangible and it guides how we speak and how we are to behave." The verb-driven Cherokee language reflects the emphasis on relationships and movement on multiple levels. It reflects four dimensions of connection: with others, with nature, with the spirit world, and with ourselves. It emphasizes the belief that we as individuals are less important than others, that the group is paramount. A simple sentence, *I see a bear*, is translated from Cherokee as *the bear, I see*, emphasizing the importance of the bear, not I, which makes complete sense if you are the one in the woods with a bear.

Sebastian Junger, in *Tribe* (2016), writes, "The word 'tribe' is far harder to define, but a start might be the people you find compelled to share the last of your food with" (xvii). He explains that tribalism is when others take responsibility for you and you are part of something much larger than yourself. This definition fits perfectly with a story Tom Belt shared about his grandparents, who had been removed to Indian Territory, now Oklahoma, in 1838. He said his father told him a story about a white family he met while going to a creek to play in 1904, before Oklahoma became a state in 1907. He said he met a man, his wife, and their five small children, who were coming down the other side of the creek in their wagon. The family was sick and needed help. He ran home to his father and told him about the white family down by the creek. His father talked with his mother and went with some other men to meet the family.

To make a long story short, Tom's grandparents gave the family their home to live in for several months, while his grandmother and other women came every day to care for the sick until they all recovered. He said the community moved his family down the road a couple of miles to a field and set up large tents there for them to live in until the white family was ready to leave. When that day came, the other Cherokee men came with their wagons and took them all back home. The white family had left and moved on to other territory farther west. He said he asked his father why they had given their entire home to people they didn't know and who were white folks in a time when white folks were not easily trusted by Native people. He said his father asked him whether he could have given his home to strangers, and Tom said he wasn't sure he could. His father said, that is just what you do. It is the Kituwah way.

Tom Belt emphasizes that this is not only doing "the Kituwah way"; this is a paradigm, a way of thinking and looking at the world. So much is riding on the ability to think and do "in the Kituwah way." It is essentially what makes someone Kituwah or Cherokee. It defines who you are as a Native person who identifies as Kituwah or Cherokee. He said,

If you can't do that then you are lying to yourself and other people. You can't call yourself Kituwah. It isn't our way to not think of the suffering of others first. It you don't, then you are not doing what's "right"! If you're a cop and see someone robbing a store and you don't stop them or do anything about it, then you're not a cop. The principle is true in being a Kituwah. If you're not conscious of the situation of others, of these things, then you're not who you say you are. Then who are you? What are you? If you're untruthful to yourself, which is the worst thing of all, you cannot be true to others. This is the beginning of internal (mental) sickness. This is connected to looking back on yourself. It puts you out of the natural world and makes you in an anomalous state that isn't real. You lose contact with reality. You do this to yourself, and this is senseless!

For example, we are lying to ourselves about the state of our environmental issues in our world. Lying about our relationship to the world makes us all sick! This is how the world works, and people do not understand it. The corporate people and the politicians don't understand this important relationship and state of mind. If you don't help the world, you bring sickness into the world. *Duyugodv'i* is the internalization of this truth, this law, that we are inextricably connected to the world. This is not a code of conduct, but a code of *thinking*. Relationships matter because there are natural laws in place. There are universal laws in place. The words for sickness, disease, and feeling bad are all about "being ill."

Tom continued, "My father's explanation makes sense to Kituwahs because that's the way the world works. Kituwahs had a clear idea of what they were doing. Again, these are universal laws that impact everyone."

Another story to emphasize his point was about attending a ceremonial stomp dance, which is held on sacred ground: "At the stomp, they were taking up a collection for someone sick. I asked the headman who it was, and he said it was for a man we all knew in the community who was a preacher who preached vehemently against our ceremony and dances. When the headman came back from putting in the hat what was a good sum of money back then, I asked him if he knew this man, and he said yes. I asked him, didn't he know that this man talked bad against us and against our church? He turned and said, 'Tom, you don't have to be a member of our church to get sick. You can be anybody and get sick. This person has children and a family.'" Tom said he then remembered his father's words, "They have children and they need help. If you can't help others, what good are you? You aren't the judge. If you do what you know is right in taking care of others, then that's all you can do."

These concepts of the importance of serving others, keeping balance in all your relationships, and being mindful of a "right way or right road" of life (*duyuk'dv'i*) are foundational in the beliefs that guide you to a healthy, balanced life of *tohi*. Many in the community feel this philosophy has in contemporary times been polarized, cast as "Indian stuff/Indian culture" in opposition to "science." We've been told, "don't go there," the Western world won't value it or even acknowledge its importance as a viable concept or law of health and wellness. As recently as two generations ago, Kituwah people would participate in traditional ceremony that guided their spiritual and physical health and well-being, with some even attending a Christian church as well, not living a conflicted existence, but fitting the two worlds together. Today, there are many Christian-converted Cherokees who see ceremony as "un-Christian" or more primitive and can't see how the two philosophies (Native science and spirituality) can fit together.

Much like other philosophies and teachings of life, it is not expected to be able to always stay on the right path. But it is the journey to stay as straight as possible that matters. "If you do get off it," said one elder, "you must recognize it and get back on it. If you stay off it, you are and will be lost. It is a matter of what is correct." He continues, "the belief of the Kituwahs is that is just life lived best in the correct way. We don't know if there is enlightenment at the end, but the best we hope for is a life lived the best way possible. We fully accept life with no fear. *Duyuk'dv'i* lessens the fear. That's why old people can just walk away when there isn't any more to do. It is settled in their minds that the next world or next level is waiting, and they have no fear."

In visiting the ancient place of the Cowee Mound in Macon County, North Carolina, Tom spoke of how this site has a prominent place in Cherokee history and cosmography. Located on the Little Tennessee River, it was known as a place of commerce and trade. Tom looks at this place, where once his people prospered, before the Rutherford and Grant expeditions burned crops to the ground and ran out the inhabitants, before disease and starvation marked the transition of the land to white settlers. Instead he is reminded of how the DNA and bones of his ancestors who lived and died here became a permanent witness and resident of this ancient land, this land that is once again in possession of the Cherokee people.

Chapter Five

◇◇◇◇◇◇◇◇◇◇◇◇◇◇◇◇◇◇◇◇◇◇

INDIGENIZING COUNSELING

We are in the water together and together
we will take this journey to wholeness.

THOMAS N. BELT

Tom Belt also talks about language as medicine. He says, "The words for medicine (*nv wo ti*, Ɵ·ᏌᎫ) and to heal somebody (*ka nv wo di*, ᎤᏴᎫᏠ) are closely tied to the word for law (*di ka nv wa dv sdi*, ᏗᏲᏀᏟᎰᏗᎫ). To heal is in the word law, meaning that which you go by to heal. It represents the concept of healing and makes it into a method. It becomes law; therefore, law is a method of healing. So, laws also mean medicine, and both have a message of healing. Laws are supposed to be used to heal and are used to keep you on the road or right path. Health of mind, body, family, community, and world are bound by laws of service, concern, and mindfulness of others and our relations in the natural world around us." We are all interconnected, and what we do, think, and say affect all others. These are laws of cause and effect. In other Native traditions it is said that even the tone of our voice can change the composition of tangible objects and maybe more importantly can inject good or bad spirits in others when we speak. This makes sense as it is thought that breath is sacred.

Most anything Cherokee must come from the community first—inside to outside. Tom referred to aniKituwah (ᎠᏂᏳᏍᎦᏴ) as "one town," beginning from within the community. Cherokee belief is that individuals become stronger as they solidify more with one another as a community. Western psychology does not always understand this cultural value and its power to heal. To become "human" is to be a part of the solution in human suffering— to serve others, support others, and address the needs of others. In discussing the focus on relationships linguistically, Cherokee speakers say that what English speakers refer to as responsibility is just what should come to you in life's journey, this white path or right path of *tohi* (health/wellness). This makes sense because the language comes from a society in which the group shoulders whatever comes together. In talking about this, one elder said, "We have always been a problem-solving culture. We know bad stuff is going to happen, and we just have to figure it out as we go, but we will do it together. Oftentimes this occurred at our ceremonial grounds. This was a place where anger and problems were addressed." Anthropologist Albert Wahrhaftig's (1970) fieldwork among the Cherokee Nation in the 1950s and 1960s focused in large part on those attending stomp dances, churches, and ceremonies. He noted that many who attended were lawyers, teachers, preachers, and traditional medicine people, but all of these people came together, speaking the same language and having the same cultural values of group, clan, and matrilineage.

One elder, speaking about being at "the grounds," said, "We were poor and struggling but not depressed. We were a community because we solved problems together. Our way of life was to wake up in the morning and be grateful for what we had and not fearing what was ahead because we knew we had to fix problems so that we could keep that way of life." He continued, "Bad stuff doesn't besmirch you, but you overcome it. Not the idea that 'life isn't fair.' It just existed, and we knew things could get bad, but we didn't see it as a burden, but instead a chance to overcome and go on because life is bigger than that. That is part of *tohi*, making good out of bad." This speaks to the resiliency of tribal members. It is a way of thinking and believing that we will continue, we will survive.

The association of well-being with the act of bringing people home was a recurring theme in the talks Tom and I had. Stories of events that historically occurred on homelands were important to repeat, particularly to younger generations, letting them know that their ancestors were still there and were a reminder to their resilience and stability. Such stories provide continuity to their culture and history and connect them with their own lineages. Many tribal elders begin any public talk by identifying their family and even naming an ancestor known to have made a specific contribution historically to the tribe. This reflects their own identity and the thread that binds clans and families together. It provides a connection to place and puts it in a historical context. These stories are not only a part of Cherokee culture and cosmography, but also a feature of most tribal nations. Cosmography is an umbrella concept that unites people from many fields to better understand the history and its importance to Cherokee people today. This concept reflects the multidimensional understanding of the land, cosmos, and epistemologies among Native people who have lived in a particular place for a substantial period of time, and is uniquely identified with a culture. It doesn't separate the people from their surroundings and knowledge about the environmental, historical, ecological, and cosmological activities that have occurred through millennia. It is part of who they are, and it is greatly valued.

The disconnection of an individual from their cosmographical epistemologies is indeed part of their disconnection from identity, from an understanding of who they are or what it means to be "Cherokee." So many Native youth who have gone through treatment or personal mental health journeys will often mention this disconnect. They question who they are, an action that is symptomatic of loss of culture, language, and understanding of place and history. For Cherokees, elders will sometimes speak of how younger generations have a hard time seeing past the "Boundary," their fifty-six thousand acres, the current home of the EBCI in western North Carolina.

The naming of the Cherokees' Qualla Boundary is itself of historical and psychological interest. "Qualla" means "Polly," the name of a woman who once lived in the area, a part of the Cherokee homeland. The "Boundary" refers to the "reservation" on which the EBCI reside. It is not a reservation as is understood in relation to other federally controlled tribal territories. The EBCI, unlike all other federally recognized tribes, purchased their own homeland not once, but on multiple occasions (see Finger 1984). It is, I think, unfortunately referred to as the "Boundary" to discern between the two types of tribally owned lands. The word *boundary* infers a barrier, a borderline or periphery. Linguistically, it limits one to a particular space. However, it also may say that this is your place and no other place is yours. In fact, the Cherokee homeland extended for millions of acres over what is today eight states. This is not only a heritage to be proud of, but a call to know these other places better. Cherokee history and culture occurred on mountains, valleys, rivers, and creeks that continue to house important towns and features of meaning. In Tennessee, for example, there are several important towns where historical elders, leaders, and events made their mark on Cherokee culture even though some of these places are today underwater from the development of lakes and dams. Nevertheless, recognizing where these places are allows a broader understanding of the influence and richness of Cherokee occupation for thousands of years. These places are an important connection to Cherokee identity.

In surrounding counties and states, the rich history and cosmography of the Kituwah people are evident. It is hard for young people to see the significance of mounds, rivers, trails, petroglyphs, and ancient turnpikes that reflect vast negotiations, trade, and diplomacy of a sovereign people. Complicating the issue of identity is the hesitancy of young adult Cherokees to learn the language. There are some who adorn themselves with signage of Indigenous culture, who are well educated and are "members in the community" yet don't feel as though the language is important or critical to the future of the people. This presents many problems, with who you are "at the core" as a major issue. It is language that identifies you as unique and perpetuates a worldview that has accumulated for millennia. As Tom Belt has said many times, "Cherokee language is more than a code for English."

Many would also argue that this disconnect would include, even more importantly, the spiritual identity that shapes the heart of young people. In a recent meeting of speakers, we were reminded that the Cherokee word for "thought" is closely related to the word for "heart." In this discussion, elders were speaking to the endemic presence of drugs and violence, which are killing their children and jeopardizing their communities and their future. One of the first statements to be made was "our hearts need to heal." The speaker continued, "This problem of addiction can't be 'treated' with other drugs or expensive programs, because this is a spiritual problem. Indian people carry the experiences of their parents and grandparents. With them, the language that allows them to impart what is happening to them in the world is being lost." The language *is* their identity but also is the way in which they could explain what was happening to their families and communities. The loss of language is synchronous with loss of place and spirituality. The speaker finished his thought by saying, "With this loss of identity is a people who become hollow, and this hollowness can only be filled with place and identity, which equals our spirituality." Another speaker commented, "We have forgotten our places. Who we are was how we lived here, our way of life. Loss of gardens, loss of how we gathered plants—this is a way of life we identified with and is another indication of our loss of identity."

There is much concern for future generations of Cherokee people. Assimilation, modernization (obsession with videos, technology-centered entertainment, smartphones), an abrupt change in diet (within the last two to three generations), and the physical and mental health issues that come with these changes present real and present dangers for Native communities. Native psychologist Joseph P. Gone (Gros Ventre) urges providers to trust in the power of ancient culture and epistemologies that have supported Indigenous peoples for thousands of years. Gone's keynote presentation at Western Carolina University's Rooted in the Mountains Symposium in 2017 was titled "Recovering Indigenous Knowledge Traditions for Rethinking Mental Health." He provided examples of how Native "culture is treatment" by discussing the development of programs within his tribe, the Gros Ventre, using "traditional stories, cosmological knowledge, games, and ceremonial protocols that created reality, circulated generative power, and neutralized destructive power for [his] community." He explained that by collecting traditional stories and protocols, he "uncovered subjugated Indigenous knowledge" and documented cultural psychologies that existed for his people. He provides a methodology and practice that can be used for other tribes in their own journeys to healing.

Addiction is always present in discussion of current health issues that face Native communities. In a meeting of elders and clinicians in the Cherokee community, one tribal member who had experienced the pain of addiction in his family felt that the issue of being disconnected was real and central to the discussion. He said, "Addiction is insular in that it keeps you apart from everything—your family, your loved ones, your culture." Another speaker said that addiction is akin to being obsessed: "Our old people used to say that obsession takes you away from reality. You can't be *tohi* because it makes you out of balance."

A study by psychologist Bruce Alexander in the 1970s provided a much-needed expanded view of addiction. Rats were given the choice of a steady diet of heroin-laced water or a rat "utopia," parks that contained a plethora of opportunities for them to socialize, play, and have sex. They ignored the addictive water and instead readily chose to engage in their "rat park" with others. Journalist Johann Hari summarized Alexander's study in his 2015 book *Chasing the Scream*. Writing in the *Guardian* about his book, Hari (2016) concluded that "the opposite of addiction is not sobriety. The opposite of addiction is connection. And our whole society, the engine of our society, is geared towards making us connect with things, not people."

This idea of connection is also central to Indigenous ways of thinking. It is our connections that affect the behavior, expectations, and decisions that ultimately have bearing on our health and well-being.

For colonized people, the whole thrust of assimilation was to embrace and internalize those values of the dominant society that might allow them to survive. It was dominated by the idea of individualism, and later the unfortunate application of social Darwinism, "survival of the fittest," which influenced many industrialists and politicians at the turn of the nineteenth and twentieth centuries. It was used to rationalize everything from imperialism and racism to child labor.

Because ideas of colonialization, imperialism, and assimilation help justify separation and discrimination, as well as the hierarchical thinking that has been attributed to the Y chromosome (see Tannen 2007), it is often taken for granted that the notion of tribalism or interconnectedness is a naive or primitive way of thinking. However, as we face serious social and climatological issues, many experts are urging us to think in a more holistic and interconnected way for the sake of both humanity and the planet. Similarly, inclusivity is the major buzzword of the twenty-first century as we encourage more of it in education, the workplace, health care, and the environment.

To return to the topic of addictions: an issue that has been too long under-funded and undersupported in Native communities is the critical need for culturally appropriate and tribally unique substance abuse treatment and af-tercare for youth. Historically, treatment options have included matrix mod-els, twelve-step models, biological models, chemical models, choice models, and "just say no" models, but what models have we ignored because they didn't come from a pharmaceutical company, or from a Western perspec-tive? Let's consider instead an approach to helping one become *tohi* again, an approach that comes from older ways of thinking, prioritizing the care and teaching of one person by another or the value of connecting to a larger family and community system. Instead of the "rugged individualism" of our dominant culture, let's consider the value of a sense of shared identity, cul-ture, language, and beliefs that re-instill a sense of self-worth and belonging.

One of the national goals to improve the health of American citizens is aimed at closing a number of health disparity gaps for disadvantaged pop-ulations, including American Indians and Alaska Natives. This goal is spe-cifically highlighted in the 2014 *Native Youth Report*, a report and call to ac-tion from President Obama (EOP 2014). Among the unmet health needs for many American Indian and Alaska Native communities is the lack of per-manent culturally appropriate mental health treatment resources for youth. Funding for these programs has been referred to as a patchwork, with lit-tle opportunity or financing to develop evaluation components to measure long-term outcomes or add promising strategies for more comprehensive interventions.

A 2006 study of mental health in the United States concluded that Native American youth have more problems than any other group and experience higher rates of anxiety, substance abuse, and depression (Olson and Wahab 2006). Even more telling is the fact that among Native adolescents in some communities, suicide rates are thirteen times higher than among the general US population (Ballard et al. 2015). These compelling numbers illustrate an urgent need for increased resources and a more comprehensive approach to understanding the scope and variability of problems involved.

Native treatment centers, particularly federal youth treatment centers, have historically relied on an overwhelmingly higher number of non-Native counselors and Western-oriented programming and counseling materials to treat Native youth. So the norm in counseling among Native populations is pretty similar to other methodologies used in counseling settings through-out the United States. This includes placing models used for middle-class white children on Native adolescents, with pan-Indian elements justifying "culturally appropriate" treatment. I have worked with counselors for many years and have been perplexed by the absence of tribally specific language, culture, and trauma-respondent models. Some approaches have seemed to be antithetical to cultural values.

To provide some examples of how off the mark Western counseling protocols are, the following are common realities for Native youth in treatment. A large majority began smoking before the age of ten. Many of these young people suffered multiple deaths of parents, grandparents, aunts, uncles, cousins, and close friends, often witnessing those deaths themselves. An overwhelming majority suffered sexual and physical abuse from very young ages; most abusers were people they knew. Often they would be left with few to no role models or mentors who could help them mediate the multiple layers of trauma that had been perpetrated on them. And far too many dropped out of school in their freshman or sophomore year because they saw no future or began to have suicidal ideations by the time they finished elementary school.

To compound the stigmas and inappropriate treatment of these youth, Western models seem to be more punitive and critical than understanding and healing. What follows are evaluations of patients as authored by psychologists working with Native youth. These evaluations do not reflect a single individual but have been generalized to reflect common responses, in most cases to young people who are very familiar with death, abuse, trauma, neglect, abandonment, and poverty:

> The profile of this young person is characterized by negativism, overt hostility, and mistrust of others, combined with an edgy defensiveness against criticism and the efforts to deny underlying feelings of dejection and self-condemnation. Fearing domination and brutalization, the client assumes a socially provocative if not overtly aggressive public posture, reflecting a belief that only alert vigilance and vigorous counteraction can obstruct the malice of others. Although there is a desire to be close to others, there is a fear of displaying this weakness, and a struggle ensues to keep melancholy feelings from public view.

> The client's public posture of being a cold and defiant teenager springs from generalized animosity toward authorities and family. Moreover, there is a wish to vindicate past humiliation and grievances.

> Profile is characterized by an inflated yet insecure sense of self-worth, a defensiveness against anticipated criticism, provocative peer and family behavior, indifference to the interests and needs of others, and a seductive and self-seeking social manner. More disputatious and abrasive tendencies may ultimately exasperate and anger others. Actions such as disregarding social conventions and the rights of others may be indicative of a deficient social conscience, possibly evident in drug use, alcoholism, and sexual acting out.

At times this teenager may be devious and overtly defiant. Wary of the motives of others and often feeling unfairly treated, may be easily provoked to irritability and anger. A thin facade of sociability gives way readily to antagonistic and caustic comments, and vindictive gratification is often obtained by humiliating others. A history of sexual excesses and abandoned school and family responsibilities may be evident. Lacking deep feelings of loyalty, the client may cleverly scheme beneath a veneer of social conformity. A guiding principle is that of outwitting others, exploiting them before they exploit you. Carrying a chip on the shoulder attitude, readily attacking those whom he/she distrusts.

Has little or no compassion for others and believes that they cause their own problems by being weak.

Is hedonistic and exploitive, finds rules restrictive, questions convention and conformity, and occasionally has problems with authorities. That drug use and other delinquent activities fit recreational patterns of stimulus seeking and narcissistic indulgence is likely.

So is this the manner in which we diagnose and respond to young people who have lived with extensive trauma, abandonment, and violence? Do we relegate them to a continuous and perpetual system of naming and labeling that will follow them throughout their lives, a system that they themselves do not relate to or understand? Where within this model do we see a hint of empathy, humaneness, or cultural sensitivity? It is imperative that the behavioral health and medical community understand that our paradigm regarding treatment of Native youth needs to change. The models used in Western counseling most often do not align with Indigenous values or epistemologies. As Eduardo Duran advocates, stop the psychobabble and begin to understand where these young people are in their own struggle to be whole again. And within all of this, we, as a society, still need to recognize the long-term implications of childhood trauma. There are many connections with what is experienced in our personal history and generational histories, between biology, physiology, and genetics. Epigenetics holds the lens for our families historically and gives us vision for our future. This intersection between the environmental and biological elements that make us who we are is unfortunately a model that not all of our health professionals are aware of, yet it is critical in understanding health and chronic disease, particularly if trauma and stress are part of our intergenerational experience.

As the literature continues to show, childhood trauma is one of the most important and pervasive public health concerns in American society today. It sets the stage for not only social pathologies and mental health issues, but also serious chronic diseases that bend the economic back of health-care systems. Coupled with what is known and what we are understanding about social determinants of health, childhood trauma is the critical element in the formula for how to address the many issues we face. We must learn to not blame the victim but instead offer compassion and rationale for why people self-medicate, utilize survival skills that are unhealthy for relationships, and live with the albatross of shame and fear that can underlie so many of our life decisions and maladaptive yet common behavior. Much like the roles that are taken on in dysfunctional family systems and that affect relationships throughout our lives if not understood, traumatic childhood experiences can shape our behavior and affect our physiology in ways that may not manifest critically until well into adulthood, but for many young people, problems like addiction, self-mutilation, and mental health issues may appear earlier.

What we understand from Native adolescents who have gone to treatment is that they are more likely to have high adverse childhood experience (ACE) scores, a standard measurement in trauma assessment. They are more likely to have only one parent in the home, to have experience with sexual, physical, and/or emotional abuse from a young age, to have less connection with their language, cultural beliefs, or ceremony, and to have issues with their Indian identity.

The critical question, then, is how do we treat this diverse group of young people who seem to have the highest need for treatment that is relevant, that can reconnect them with their culture and heritage, and that provides them with the self-esteem and hope that will sustain them through difficult years of transitioning from childhood to adulthood?

Even if they successfully complete a treatment program, many have to return to the dysfunctional system that sent them there because aftercare programs are virtually nonexistent and have been historically underfunded by federal or tribal governments.

In an article titled "Keeping Culture in Mind," Joseph P. Gone (2004) urges us to ground mental health service and delivery in local and community concepts. Seek out those in your community who can explain tribal epistemologies through language use and behavioral protocols. Ask about Indigenous concepts of self, personhood, behavior, healing, thought, and cosmology.

We need a revolution of sorts in the world of counseling Native youth. Having worked with Native communities on diabetes prevention, addiction, contemporary issues of Indian fatherhood, PTSD, and community health training, I have been convinced that the dominant society tends to silo these issues and that most Western-derived models just aren't effective in Native communities.

The challenge is for us to stand up and change our way of thinking, change our way of looking at problems and issues that have plagued Indian country for hundreds of years. We need to embrace an older way of understanding the relationships and dynamics of humans in this world, not only with other people, but with other species, with natural resources, with the air, with the water, with the mountains and deserts, with those places where they find refuge and strength and hope and healing, where their spirit and trust are found in ways that most of us could never imagine.

In the Cherokee community, it has been interesting to find out what traditionalists and Native speakers perceive to be the critical elements in working with youth who are trying to become whole and well once again. Tom Belt reflected on his years working with Native youth and addictions: "What our young people need more than anything is love and nurturing. They need someone to trust, someone they can rely on to be with them. I didn't ask anything from them, unlike most of their past experiences. I know that when we connected and they found we had a relationship of trust, I remember them being young people who were kind, caring, and generous. I treated them as a young tribal member, identifying them with their tribe. A connection was made and they began to know who they were."

Working with linguists and speakers to better understand these concepts in a tribally specific context isn't a fast project, but it is enlightening and critical. In most of these conversations, certain themes reoccur. In the Cherokee epistemology those who are lost or who feel a sense of loss have a sense of inconsistency and direction; all is "askew." As Tom has said, those young and old who are "depressed," for example, are—in Cherokee terms—looking inward toward themselves and not outward as Kituwahs have always done. Those who have become out of balance have, in Tom's terms, "fallen off the white path or right path. Elders taught that there was happiness and safety on that road, and it was part of our science, the natural law."

It was also mentioned that in the historical record, an early traveler into Cherokee territory had written that there were no orphans or paupers in Cherokee society. According to tribal law and tradition, one's kinship, language, and identity made sure they were never alone or without. In other words, everyone had a place, they belonged, everyone was part of something. In today's society, we often compartmentalize orphans and paupers and place them outside of relationships, outside of community. One elder said that "non-Natives don't understand the concept of tribalism—being part of something larger than yourself. Tribalism is ultimately about being connected. Having a sense of place. This is translated in the language, as it allows one to trust the natural order again, the right path, to be the way you are supposed to be. Safety and empowerment comes from that."

Native psychologist Joseph P. Gone (2017) speaks of the quest to understand the ancestral concepts of the power of thought. He asks tribal people to think about and inquire of elders about teachings regarding the supernatural power of thought. For example, in the Cherokee language the word for "thought" (*a da na te di*, DⱢθႱꞀ, to think about) has the same root as the word for "heart" (*a da na to gi*, DⱢθVУ): thought comes from your heart. Tom emphasizes the importance of this connection: "The Western world encourages people to separate the body, to prioritize the mind or intellect over that intrinsic part of us that makes us empathize, feel compassion, or even shows how emotion can make us sick. It is often the heart that connects one to their ancestry and the spirit that lives on from them." There are places in tribal communities where one can sense the presence of others, those who lived there long, long ago. I have heard from many who visited sites in Kituwah country that they immediately felt that presence and felt the comfort of hundreds of others.

It is near these places where often ceremony continues to bridge time. It provides the backdrop of peace and comfort for those participating in ritual that has identified people for who they are. Ceremony is a major part of their whole health. It provides balance to the individual and continuity for all who come regularly and participate, even as it also comes with the responsibility to remember and perpetuate these experiences that provide identity and meaning. By performing ritual or protocols, we internalize the meaning intended with these actions and associate it with the experiences we have in ceremony. When I was a child, it was the teaching of my mother's church to conduct a foot-washing ritual during an annual holy day. The action of washing someone's feet was intended to teach humility and service. The performance internalized the meaning, and I remember it to this day. And for those who worship literally in nature, place can add a layer of meaning and connection to ceremony.

Tom speaks of the importance of ceremony: "Ceremony is simply a reminder of what is true. It is a reminder of responsibility and order—the right time and place. It involves protocols and reflects a 'natural science' of order. There is not a ceremony that does not remind us of place. What is important in the cycle of life, we remind ourselves daily through these rituals. Without this, we would be like you and it all would be dead."

One elder said, regarding Western diagnoses, "Disease models often relieve a person from any responsibility (I mean you can't blame a person for being sick). In the old ways, you had to do what you were told—your health was a partnership with the medicine person to become whole again. When you make a choice to get back on the road again, when you do that, then everyone will help. Ceremony is important, but you can't waste it. It is done when the medicine person knows absolutely that the person seeking help will comply. Ceremony is to be repeated. It is a way to keep you from being lost. It is the power of thought and spirit. When all are together, we have *tohi*."

Another said, "You aren't given a map by a healer. They are on the journey with you! They go where you are and take time to talk about these concepts with elders. They provide more than just advice; they know you need groundwork in understanding. They say, 'we are going to do this . . . we are in the water together.' How can you trust someone if they are not with you?"

Regarding Native youth treatment, we need to support, fund, and encourage a change in how counseling models are developed. Energy, money, and direction should follow the advice of Native scholars like Gone and Duran, and tribal elders who have more than twelve thousand years of accumulated traditional and ecological knowledge, to invest in tribally specific understandings of how to reconnect youth to a larger family, identity, and place. Federal and philanthropic agencies need to fund more tribally specific and linguistically appropriate treatment models, including support for aftercare and intergenerational, tribally cosmographic models honoring the traditional tribal landscape and healing it provides. Tribes need to urgently invest in their language speakers and work with them to develop healing models based on the science that has been preserved for centuries within the language.

To exemplify how different these paradigms are for non-Natives: in an informal conversation, a person who was empathetic to the overwhelming problems of substance abuse among the Kituwah people as reflected in local news asked me, "What *is* the answer? . . . Why has there been such mediocre success with reducing the problem of alcohol abuse, opioid addiction, and other related substance abuse problems in their community?" My response, which I don't think was fully understood, or may have been too simple, was, "because we don't value the healing power of their language and culture, and we expect them to deal with these issues like we do in a colonized world, without ceremony and connection to their ancestors."

Those Native youth for whom language or culture is not accessible should be given the chance to learn about their heritage in their healing process. This is a great opportunity for intergenerational work with elders who can help them learn about language, culture, and ceremony. They can assist not only young clients, but counselors and staff who will be working with those young people who are seeking healing.

We need to stand up and change our way of thinking about treatment modalities. It's about healing the wounds of multigenerational trauma, it's about connecting with lives and families, and it's about finding hope, emotional bonding, and the value of lives. It's about the little ones that are tied by biology and soul to lineages centuries old in a place that gives them balance and strength and hope. It is about the core, intrinsic value of belonging and being part of something larger than oneself. Instead, our "health-care" system is ultimately about money, politics, and bureaucracy. Anyone who has experience with youth mental health and substance abuse treatment knows well that adolescent treatment and aftercare has never been a priority, has always been considered too costly, only possible if there was enough grant money available, and has only ever been thought of as an extraneous appendage to treatment.

Chapter Six

⬥⬥⬥⬥⬥⬥⬥⬥⬥⬥⬥⬥⬥⬥⬥⬥⬥

WE ARE *OF* THIS PLACE

Integrating Traditional Science and Health

> Rooted is a word that in Cherokee means helper. It is
> more than the roots just helping the tree stand up and
> live, but it encompasses how the tree aids the life of
> all that surrounds it. It reflects a system of giving.
>
> THOMAS N. BELT

Over the last decade at Rooted in the Mountains, ever since our first symposium in 2010, we have listened to Native scientists (including many lay community members) and Western-trained scientists discuss how we can utilize traditional knowledge to provide a broader and often clearer lens to understand our place in the world and to address our contemporary problems.

As we have tackled issues of mountain destruction, misuse and abuse of water, the interconnection of health and land, spiritual and natural laws of Native people that guide behavior and address social issues, plants for food and medicine, and sacredness of land and place, among other topics, we are reminded year after year by the Native speakers and elders that all these issues, like the Cherokee language, reflect—and reflect on—the quality and dynamics of relationships. Relationships are at the core of our existence. We feel the vitality of life being connected with others, and that doesn't only include other humans. There is a growing body of literature that shows how much just being outside, with what the Lakota refer to as "all my relations," can improve our attitude and sense of well-being. The trees, plants, streams, rivers, and even tiny animals going about their business can provide us with a sense of calm and *ulilohi'* (ᏋᏟᎰᎥ): things happening as they are "supposed to be," life surrounding us and we a part of "it." The healing that comes from knowing we are a part of something much larger than ourselves can be significant.

Connecting the thought of being in the forests with health, both physical and mental, reinforces current research. Mohab Ibrahim from the University of Arizona shared his story in a short interview on National Public Radio in December 2019. His brother was experiencing headaches and found that when he visited his garden they would subside. Ibrahim followed up by conducting research with rats and green light and found that, indeed, there was a positive relationship between pain reduction and exposure to the color green. Other stories of patients being exposed to green light and experiencing pain reduction were also a part of this story. Many who find working in their gardens or hiking in forests healing would agree that there is a direct correlation between exposure to the color green and feeling better.

Tom says the Cherokee word for green is *a tse i* (ᏗᎥᎢ), which is symbolic of rebirth and health. The closely related word *i tse i* (ᏔᎥᎢ) means "new"; he saw immediately how the color green for plants and light could alleviate depression and pain and be health related. He went on to explain, "When we say the mountains and plants and water and all of the life therein is an intrinsic part of us, [we mean] this power of color, which is reflected in life all around us, is something we can feel. It becomes a part of you, and you become a part of it. You can feel that connectedness in your soul. It is as deep and pervasive as you can verbalize, and it makes sense that when you damage and exploit these places, you feel that as well. This further makes the case that for real mountain people, like your mother, we share those feelings and values just as Kituwahs." Tom went on to explain that words for colors have an *i* (a long *e* sound) at the end of each word, and this is a syllable that is used for water, reflecting a liquid. He says that both colors and music are represented as liquid.

Broad international research has concluded that outdoor environments or "green spaces" improve health-related quality of life and reduce stress. Researchers in Japan note that "forest bathing" (*shinrinyoku*) can "contribute to a decrease in mortality due to cancers in Japan" (Cheng et al. 2009). In an article titled "A Doctor Explains How to Take Advantage of the Healing Powers of Nature," Eva Selhub (2021) includes these studies to talk about her own experiences as a physician responding in positive physiological and psychological ways to the beauty and wonders of nature. Even though these findings are wonderful and exciting, I would venture to say that most rural-living people already knew these things. For sure, Indigenous peoples have had this understanding for millennia, and these ideas are firmly ensconced in their minds. Why has it taken so long for Westerners to get it? My opinion is that arrogance and ego have placed people at the center of the universe, while other species—and even other non-White people—are seen as inferior or undervalued. This egocentrism has been illustrated by contrasting Cherokee and many other Indigenous languages with English. In Cherokee, for example, if you see or want something, you note the object before you talk about it: *ama agwaduliha* (**DᎣ DᏗᏍᏆᎤᏈ**) means "water, I want," as opposed to English, in which one would say, "I want water." This expresses the order of importance. In Cherokee very rarely does a sentence start with oneself.

It has been noted by Cherokee linguists that one's egocentrism can be understood in the way one speaks, indicating where one's place is in the universe. This is clear even in a movie such as *Little Big Man* (1970), which depicts fairly accurate elements of Native culture: the chief that is teaching Dustin Hoffman's character about Native ways comments that white men think that everything is dead because the way they speak reflects their own lack of consciousness. Chief Dan George, who acted against Hoffman in the film, also added, "If you talk to animals, they will talk with you and you will know each other. If you do not talk with them, you will not know them and what you do not know, you will fear. What one fears, one destroys" (George and Hirnschall 2003, 32).

History is rife with early Contact accounts that reflect a belief (not just an attitude) that non-European people were savages, primitives, and un-human. The consequences amounted to the largest genocide in human history: an estimated sixty to eighty million Amerindians died during the era of Contact (Stannard 1992a, 1992b). Many works available today provide the shocking details of torture and death for a substantial percentage of the Native population not long after Contact. *Salvation and the Savage* by Robert Berkhofer (1965), *In Defense of the Indians* by Bartolomé de Las Casas ([1550] 1992), *Ethnic Cleansing and the Indian* by Gary Clayton Anderson (2014), and *Exterminate Them!* by Clifford E. Trafzer and Joel R. Hyer (1999) are only a few titles of many that provide insight into the horrors of watching one's people be brutally exterminated en masse. This idea is so prevalent that the phrase "merciless Indian savages" was written into the Declaration of Independence! Ironically, the declaration was written during a decisive period of a few years when the Cherokees were attacked in a simultaneous assault by four "state" militias, an event that proved decisive in marginalizing the Cherokee presence as a geopolitical force to westward expansion (Wunder 2000).

It is difficult to wrap our minds around the significant number of human lives lost, not to mention the wholesale slaughter of thousands of animals and decimation of tons of plants, both understood as sacred in Indigenous cultures. The horrors of exploitation and colonization are so unimaginable that the extreme ways in which these acts altered the world forever defy our grasp. In speaking of this, Tom Belt mentioned how Cherokee language contextualized this mindset and these historical behaviors:

In this time of the COVID-19 pandemic, we would use the word *sque sta ud'sgwisda* (ᏅᎶᏫᏖᎶᎥ) to indicate that there is a lot (of stuff) and in this case sickness. Another word for reference to even greater volume of something (e.g., feelings, loneliness, pain) would be *u tsa ta* (ᏅᎬᏫ), used to identify intensity—something that is so bad now that we are responsible for doing something about it. It becomes like a medical term "code blue," saying that this is real serious and something is really severe or extreme and needs immediate attention. But when talking about the most extreme level of meanness, the word *u ne gu tsa da* or *ta* (ᏅᏁᎫᏨᎶ, he or she is mean) is *une ga* (ᏅᏁᎦ, white) *utsa ta* (ᏅᎬᏫ, volume of intensity). This is a "post-Columbian" Cherokee word referencing colonialism. That feeling or action is "intensely white" or over-the-top mean. So, *une gu tsa da* (ᏅᏁᎫᏨᎶ) = a meanness that came with colonialism.

The extreme measures of meanness and evil such as population decimation, disease, and loss of culture, land, language, economy, and matrilineality all came to them through white invasion, encroachment, exploitation, assimilation, and colonization. All were unthinkable prior to European invasion.

Well-documented European notions of the primitive and savage nature of Indigenous peoples have rationalized various Indian policies that have jeopardized Indigenous health and well-being since the first treaties were signed. We still ignore the horrendous decisions and policies that have been made, from attempts at total eradication of Native peoples to the elimination of their culture and language (e.g., through boarding school policy), which hold for them the science that allowed them great physical and mental health for millennia (for a reasonable and enlightening discussion of these events, see Jones 2004).

This Western arrogance, of course, lent itself to also devaluing the sophistication of knowledge that Indigenous people possessed. It is only now, more than five hundred years after Contact, that Western science is learning from Indigenous peoples. A recent example would be the collaboration between the Diné or Navajo Nation and NASA in the study of how the universe began (Bartels 2019). In this partnership Western scientific knowledge and cultural or Indigenous science have equal footing. Astrobiologist Daniella Scalice says, "There is no difference between traditional cultural ways of generating knowledge and the ones that science uses." This is a far cry from the colonizing paradigms espoused at the turn of the twentieth century by health professionals who saw all Native knowledge as "primitive."

What might extend our thinking about sacredness, natural laws, and Native science is the notion of spirituality. There is no word for spirituality in Cherokee; instead, there is a reference to the science of the consciousness of all that is around us being alive and having spirit. For the Western concept of faith, Kituwahs can only come close by use of *go hi ti* (ᎠᎯᏗ, belief). But when you turn it back around, it translates as "we believe it to be that way." A way to exemplify what is meant is a story of a group of young people who went to a pueblo, and the headman there told the visiting children that the morning song brought up the sun, and the evening song allowed the sun to set every day. One of the children, critical of this explanation, asked how that could be. The Pueblo elder calmly responded that "it hasn't failed us in thirty thousand years, and so we are afraid to stop this ritual each morning and evening." Tom says, "There is no intrinsic way to really explain that in a Western way. We are just acknowledging the science of the rise and set of the sun each day and giving it the proper respect it deserves." He continues, "It doesn't mean anything to you. It's just a rise and setting of the sun. We understand it as something sacred. We acknowledge it as a scientific fact and honor that with ceremony."

Things, therefore, are supposed to be done in a certain way, a natural way that recognizes the spirit of all that surrounds us and is in the universe. In 1998 NASA buried partial remains of geologist Eugene Shoemaker on the moon in lunar soil. Because his remains were placed on the moon, many tribal people believe that the moon is no longer "clean," but it has been soiled by death. The importance of this to their cosmological beliefs cannot be overstated. Tom said, "The first question that might come to mind is what gives you the right to do that? The right to contaminate that which Creator has provided to us for life? It is, again, arrogance and ego that puts us out of contact, out of our relationship with the natural world. We have changed something that we have no right to change, and it remains altered permanently. It is this permeance that is the grand gesture that is made which impacts all of humanity forever. The moon was used in reverence and with purpose. Now it is a cemetery."

In effect it becomes a monument to arrogance. There is no singular word for science in Cherokee, but it can be described as and is related to the word for belief. The same is said for spirituality, what people have called superstition. We now agree with Indigenous peoples that their beliefs have value. The greatest difference may be that Native science has a conscience. If you create nuclear waste, knowing what you are doing, that is not having a conscience. The money, power, and energy used in creating waste that takes millennia at best to go away does not justify keeping the lights on, says one elder from Oklahoma. Its presence has caused so many deaths, birth defects, and disruptions to the ecology of our world. Saving even one life, one child from a lifetime of physical ailments, is that not enough to justify the elimination of hazardous waste? It is dark thinking to rationalize health and lives for profit.

However, in talking about keeping the lights on, Tom's father commented that he didn't understand why most people were afraid of the dark. Fire, according to Kituwah belief, is animate—a living being that gives light and warmth. Heat is energy, a natural element. In today's world, night doesn't exist for everyone. For many people who live in or near major metropolitan areas, light pollution interferes with connection and recognition of the celestial beings, those relatives in which we share our composition. Maybe a reason why most southeastern tribal peoples held their ceremonies at night was that night was a sacred time. Stories were told to children; dances and music were made alongside the fire, under the stars. Tom reminds me that "Kituwahs only dance at night. Maybe Creator sees us better at night because we point up and say it's not dark up there. We send our prayers to Creator. It reminds us where we are in the universe, not just here on earth, and if you understand that, you can understand science. When you see a star at night, it makes you realize how small we are. We are supported by that tree you stand near. It doesn't ask from us, but instead gives to us. They are benevolent and help us, and all they ask is that we leave them alone."

Mohawk leader Katsi Cook (2018) has said that plants will come all the way to your doorstep to help you, further evidence that we are all in this life together. The cosmos reminds us of the vastness of life. How, then, can we think we are the center of the universe? The immediate gift of this line of thinking, that we are all part of life in this universe together, is it gives you courage and understanding that fosters a lack of fear. You know who you are, what you are connected to, and that we are *all* in this together.

It takes humility to truly understand how little we really know about the complexity of how things work and how we are connected. For example, if you work and live with Tom for any length of time, the conversation will ultimately go back to horses. He grew up with horses and worked with horses for much of his life. They are in his heart and soul. He said, "We can spend our entire lives with horses and still not know everything about them. The more we learn about horses, the more we learn about what is sacred." He relayed a story he learned from cowboy Guy Weeks, who told him the Blackfeet believe that water is alive, but if something happens to it, it can die or it can be asleep. It can kill you or it can make you lazy. A horse blows on water before it drinks. They can discover if the water is dead or asleep, and if it is so, they will not drink it. The science becomes more understandable, then, even to a white cowboy from Pecos, Texas. Tom said, "I saw a horse staring at a crow and the crow staring back at the horse. I asked Guy what that was about, and he said the horse was talking to his ancestors. Horses are born of the wind and have something in common with the crows. When they are in a full run their feet are off the ground, in space, in flight. A bird is like that. In evolutionary terms, they are indeed related. That is science. Our relationship with horses is based on trust. It is a tangible thing. It is a reciprocal relationship that can be life changing. A horse will sacrifice its life to save the one they love. There is something extremely healthy about that. The Crow people say when you're riding on a horse, you see the shadow on the ground, and you can see then, the horse allows you to be in the heavens and asks nothing in return. That is indeed a special and sacred relationship."

Related to spirituality, various Cherokee concepts for what elders call "natural laws" reflect the connection between how one lives their life as a Kituwah and the identity and meaning that it provides. As mentioned, to be a "human being" one must follow the right path, *duyuk'dv'i*. This seems a very difficult task as colonization began to take huge gouges out of Cherokee epistemology at Contact. How can one remain loyal to their identity as Kituwah, embracing traditional cultural values and "natural laws" of maintaining harmonious relationships while being assimilated into a society whose cultural values demanded the antithesis: the creation of social classes, accumulation of wealth, and transference to men of critical roles that women held for millennia regarding clan identity, ownership of property, and governance?

A case in point involves the Cherokee man Major Ridge, who was a successful plantation owner in north Georgia. He was one of the three original signers of the fraudulent Treaty of New Echota, also known as the Removal Treaty of 1835. According to Cherokee people and scholars, it was an act of suicide to sign the lands of the Cherokee people away to the government, for others to move the Kituwah people from their homeland. West, the direction of Removal, was considered the direction of death. So how could a "successful" Cherokee like Ridge commit such a reprehensible act, which caused unimaginable pain and suffering for so many people, the effects of which are still felt today? He signed the treaty knowing that he would die as a result—and indeed he did.

Tom suggested that Major Ridge, a wealthy slaveowner, had "forgotten who he was." He had become lost. He had submitted to a way of life and thought from the colonizing society. He transgressed the law of *du yu go dv hi*, a physical and spiritual law. He created an anomaly by his thoughts and actions. "An action such as this reflects that he had lost his identity as a Kituwah, a human being. He had to forgo the understanding of ancient laws that focused on our relationships with others, the land, the spirit world, and self. He was killed because he acted as a cancer and it had to be cut out." Tom continued, "Land was understood as the creation and property of someone else. It belongs to God. All that comes from it, on it, and under it is sacred."

This is an important example for many today. To forget who you are, the place from whence you come, can cause imbalance. It can separate you from those laws that direct you to *tohi*. For many elders, it is supportive relationships, service, and ceremony that bring you back to who you are meant to be. They bring you home.

In Vincent Werito's impressive chapter, "Understanding *Hozho* to Achieve Critical Consciousness: A Contemporary Diné Interpretation of the Philosophical Principles of *Hozho*" (2014), he describes the Diné thoughts on *hozho*, or living life in beauty and harmony. This work exemplifies the critical part language plays in understanding a way of life, using millennia-old traditional knowledge to explain how one follows a path I would argue is much akin to the Cherokee notion of *tohi*. He shares that this knowledge was handed down orally for generations. It is also with the Diné that an understanding of *hozho* "is a part of all traditional Navajo ceremonies and cultural teachings because of its emphasis on harmonious outcomes in most every situation" (26).

Werito notes that this philosophy is the core of the Diné way of life and way of thinking and living and that his elders taught him to "listen carefully and with purpose" (28). It is "a way of life we strive to live, yet it is also part of our thoughts, language, prayers, and songs, and is integral to our inherent human quality for making sense of our lives and striving for harmony, peace, and justice" (27).

These ways of thinking and living can also produce energy and power that can be transformative and take on metaphysical properties. This is not uncommon among Indigenous people, who have developed what are complex systems and ways of knowing through thousands of years of their own scientific inquiry. Much of these metaphysical concepts, also present in Kituwah cosmologies and epistemologies, can defy time and space, much like that of Aboriginal Dreamtime. All of this ancient knowledge is well preserved in tribal language, art, and ancient petroglyphs as English is often inadequate to explain or translate these concepts. In the Western world, it is physicists who are often most easily accessible to these discussions.

Chapter Seven

DECOLONIZING AND INDIGENIZING OUR MINDS FOR BETTER HEALTH

Tohi

> Stories tell us how to live and why we are here. We are here
> to live in the best way and with the best health we can. Our
> ancestors' stories are explaining the science of how to live.
>
> THOMAS N. BELT

The medicine of Cherokee language shows us how to live and understand our place in the world. We suffer without it. Tom says, "Our core identity as Kituwah people rests largely on our understanding of the world through the eyes of our people millennia ago. The stories that are passed down teach us who we are and how we got to be here and how to live with ourselves, others around us, and the spirit world."

As he was working with a linguist in transcribing some biblical language, Tom had several insights on the use of the word *ela na gi'* (ᏏᏇᎾᎩ) (*gi* is a transient vowel and the speaker's preference):

> *Ela nv gi*, *ela wo di'* are words suspected to translate to "everywhere" or "globally." *Elo hi ni gv i'* is contracted to *elo ni gv i*, which means "worldwide," and in the New Testament, that's the word they use for paradise. Where do those converted Cherokee speakers get *elo ni gv*? To Cherokees this was paradise. Everything we needed was here, a concept much like the Garden of Eden. As we understood in our cosmology this is our beginning place. This is where you begin as a human being, as a soul. Your job is to learn and do your best to understand what this world and this life is about. That's why plants and animals are sacred. This isn't ours. That's why we say our name is

Kituwah, which means we are people of the dirt that belongs to God. We are here to learn and live well in this dimension. You have to prepare yourself for the next life. You have to learn what sacred is and what life is. Therein lies the beginning of understanding the meaning of life and creation. It is the science of everything. The Western world categorizes it all into biology, astronomy, botany, physics, and so forth, but it's the way the world works. You are given to understand how our societies were structured to make it conducive to live the kind of life where we understood the sacredness of being here. That's what leaders, medicine men and women, and clan mothers and all of those people had accumulated over their lifetime. That's how they adjudicated things. They knew what good things were and how things fit together.

He continued, "There's another dimension as well. We understand that there are people who don't get it, don't understand how this life works. They didn't learn about how to have good relationships and how that brings health for others and ultimately yourself. They didn't 'get it,' and if they didn't, they may have done things to harm others because that isn't the way of *duyuk'dv'i*, the right way. That may mean that they have to stay here until they do 'get it,' they do learn the right way. That doesn't mean reincarnation, it just means that your time as a living organism has to end but that doesn't mean you have to leave. You have to stay here as long as it takes for you to learn what you need to learn."

Explaining further, Tom said, "So you may have encountered things that 'go bump in the night,' some may refer to them as 'evil spirits,' but we don't see them as evil, they just are lost souls trying to figure a way to make things right, and they will eventually, and get to move on as well, once they 'get it right.'"

But Tom's point from his use of the term *ela na gi'* is that this is the beginning place, and that kind of discipline and that way of looking at the world is what is expected of Kituwahs. Tom said, "We might have to help others, even in the next dimension, but they'll have more time to figure it out. They will see more clearly, hear more clearly, and eventually figure it out. Other tribes share this philosophy too. I was told the example of Cheyenne women, who, after the Battle of Little Big Horn, went up to Custer's body and drove their awls into Custer's ears so that in the next world it may help him hear. They were trying to help him make his way in the next dimension."

Tom continued, "In the Kituwah understanding, their homeland is paradise and all that they need is there. It is inclusive of *duyuk'dv'i* and abiding by the natural laws of the world. As the Cherokee stories reflect, the plants and animals were here first. They are of a higher order and knew these things. Humans came later and were assisted by the plants and animals as long as they didn't abuse that privilege of their help. But because we did, we lost the ability to communicate in language directly with them. Instead, our learning from them takes much more time and effort and curiosity on our part."

Part of decolonizing our lives includes creating a paradigm that reduces our stress. On this topic Tom again relied on lessons from speakers: "Living life without stress as our old people did, meant they were living life unafraid, not because they didn't have anything to fear. It was that our language and stories didn't teach us how to fear."

We can think of stress as another gift of colonization or disease of civilization. Results from a recent community health assessment in the EBCI community cited that 33 percent of community members reported feeling increased stress resulting in health problems. This is, to my knowledge, the first time the EBCI community identified stress as a public health issue. Health and wellness studies are rife with stress and disease connections. Stress is associated with metabolic disorders, heart disease, high blood pressure, mental health issues, and issues of early mortality.

Tom relayed the story of his attendance at a community meeting. In front of him sat two elders he knew well who were first-language speakers. One of them leaned over and spoke in Cherokee to the other, asking him what it was that the person up front was referring to that was causing such a fuss. The other elder responded that the presenter was talking about stress and the ways it could affect you. The first elder thought a minute and then again in Cherokee said, "What is it that they are afraid of?" Tom said the light bulb came on, and he realized that some elders in the community use the word "stress" synonymously with the word "fear." He thought, yes! That is it! This is that difference that he had noticed between younger generations and those older people that he had grown up with and that he often engaged with in traditional settings. There is a difference in their demeanor. That is, there is no reflection of stress in their actions, their voice, or the way they carry themselves.

When Tom was asked how Cherokees would translate the word "fear," he said that *asga e ha* (DꙡᎥᏍᏕᎥ) would refer to "harm." Something that causes harm can cause fear. He continued, "The cause of fear for Europeans was different from that of Native people in that often the cause of fear for many Europeans was the unknown, and also they feared a loss of power or control. They didn't know what might happen. The teachings of Kituwahs says do not be afraid of the unknown, the realization of your own limitations. Not knowing or *ni gol (i) gv na* (ᎲᎠᏈᎬᎠ) means they don't recognize it. There is a reason for everything, we may just not understand it. To stop whatever harms can also stop fear. If you are worried about something, you are afraid of it, but you can fix it." We can see by the verb-based language of the Cherokee that they were problem solvers. They were adapters.

In a Western way of thinking, fears or phobias would not have been a part of traditional life. My mother and the old mountains folks used to talk about how one should face their fear. I remember well, calling for her to come and take care of a snake or spider or some other issue when we were in the woods, and she would say, you shouldn't be afraid of the woods or even the night. If you understand these places or these critters or what goes on during the night, you can begin to appreciate them. If you can appreciate them, you can fix your fear. She, like many of those from whom she learned, those who have lived here for thousands of years, understood that knowing about place and what's in it and what happens is about understanding the reality of being in the mountains. The touchstone regarding reality, then, was place.

For Kituwahs, ceremony and place were interconnected. There was no fear in going to a place for ceremony because the reality was you were there to be taught and to become whole. Tom said, "For 150 years we have been told that use of our ceremonies and the experience of them in 'place' was wrong and demonic. Instead, this is where we had music, shook shells, sang, and made medicine. It becomes a decision that each person has to make to continue these traditions that are ancient. It takes courage to continue, the courage of our ancestors, to learn about the fire and water, and just how to be a real 'human being.' We've had Kituwahs who have lived their lives walking around with a big hole inside of them, and many who are learning about our traditions and language are filling that hole and being human again."

We return to the discussion Tom had while assisting a colleague in understanding the early 1800s Cherokee translation of the New Testament. He commented that there are Cherokee words used in that translation that are not used very much today, as indicated in the case of *elo ni gv* or "paradise." He had been mulling over another word, one used in a passage to indicate being a "fool." He conferred with several other speakers and said the word used was *u la sga ni s di* (ᎤᎳᏍᎨᏂᏍᏗ), meaning someone who is always angry about something, someone who is grumpy, gripey, or cranky. The language then indicates that those who are cranky and complaining or negative were considered foolish. Again the language is emphasizing the importance of quality of relationships. These people must not be thinking clearly, or their minds are murky, *ka na sa da* (ᎧᎾᏌᏓ), which means their mind is like a nest, twigs and all intermingled.

This foolishness, not thinking clearly, reflects the antithesis of Kituwah ways of being, of acting, of thinking. If you are complaining, you must then be out of harmony. Cherokee anthropologist Robert K. Thomas (1958) refers to the Cherokee value of "harmony ethic." He says that if one is in disagreement or in conflict with what is being discussed, in order to uphold the harmony ethic, one would show one's disagreement by merely getting up and leaving the discussion. This would occur in formal and informal settings. Again, the most important element of this value was maintaining the quality of relationships, illuminating their importance. This reflects both how things were done "in the right way" and how a person's disagreement was not held against them.

Tom says that three major laws of Kituwahs speak to the importance of our relationships. The first major law, *ga du gi* (ᏤᏎᎩ) sets the foundation, teaches us our mission in life, and is the mechanism for how things work. He says, "To be Kituwah was the belief in *ga du gi*, which meant for one to always look to benefit others, to join together and work together for others' benefit. It also has to do with cycles in life and ceremony, and even how biology works—things working in unison, symbiotic living. It indicates action, doing. It helps us understand our purpose as any law of science. Science connects us with all around us in the world and the universe."

Another law is *ga lv quo di* (ᏤᎸᎤᏗ), which is to care about one another, to like and respect your people. This differs from love your people, which is yet another law, *ada ge yu di* (ᎠᏓᎨᏳᏗ), which means to hold on to one another, be connected to one another. This third law refers to an emotion so deep and visceral, it is akin to emotionally embracing in such a way that you cannot let go. It reflects an extension of yourself. If they hurt, you hurt. This is also used for the concept of sacred. It involves deep benevolence. These are the words and concepts that ultimately identify one as Kituwah. Tom goes on to explain, "This is why we hold hands at ceremony, in leaving meetings and prayers, because we hold hands to the right of us and to the left of us so that we may hold one another up, and we are to go through life in this manner. This is how important our relationships are to one another, to the natural world, and to the spirit world."

This brought us back to the story of his grandfather and grandmother giving up their home to white strangers who were sick and needed a place for healing. Tom said, "I asked my grandmother why she would do such a drastic thing, and she said if we didn't do that we would be liars, we would not be the people we say we are." There is a calmness, a happiness in these words. From just looking at one word or concept of *u la sga ni s di*, Kituwahs can connect the other beliefs about *duyuktv* (ᏍᎦᎥᎢᎢ), *tohi* (ᎥᏙ), *gadugi* (ᏤᏎᎩ), *galvgwodi* (ᏤᎸᎤᏗ), and *dehigeyusesdi* (ᏍᏙᎺᏥᎦᎶᎤᏗ, you love them), which represent thousands of years of understanding how best to live in this world in peace, in love, and in happiness.

What an incredible legacy for the Kituwah people and for those who understand their language in teaching how to live this life in the best way possible. Tom, speaking of how language is medicine, often makes a point of how speaking brings you to a place of being grateful. This means one must take the time to think outward, not inward, on those things that bring happiness and thankfulness. He says that most elders are always happy and grateful to see people, for visits, for people sharing an often highly guarded commodity—time. The gratitude most often focuses on nonmaterial things and is reflected in Kituwah cultural values like service, humility, humor, and love.

Unfortunately, there are always those in today's communities who make a profession of being angry, critical, or judgmental. Tom says that this wasn't the way historically for Kituwahs, particularly elders. As mentioned, the words for thought and heart come from the same root word, *adan'dogi'*. If one is always negative or critical, their heart must not be a force for life, which it should be. Thinking is equated with the heart, and that is who you really are. If one is thinking selfishly or being greedy, the word is *ukshaleski* (ᎤᏍᎭᎴᏍᎩ, it is taken from your anus), meaning your mind is turned upside down, which is "unnatural" and out of balance because your focus is behind you (from your rear end), not forward in front of you (from your eyes). This would also include those who speak and think with their ego and pride.

For many mountain people, they too understood the direct connection between one's emotions or feelings and their status of health. In *Gunn's Domestic Medicine*, a popular medicinal guide by a physician from Knoxville, Tennessee, first published in 1830, an entire section is dedicated to the "Passions." The author, John Gunn ([1830] 1986) writes, "If you give way to the passions, you destroy the finest of the vital powers: you destroy digestion and assimilation; you weaken the strength and energies of the heart, and of the whole nervous system. The stomach is the workshop of the whole human frame and all its derangements are immediately felt in the extremities: and to prove how strongly the connection exists, between the stomach and the heart, the latter immediately ceases to beat, when the powers of the former sink and are destroyed. Distress of mind is always a predisposing cause of disease: while on the other hand, a calm and contented disposition, and a proper command over our passions and affections, are certain to produce consequences which operate against all predisposing cause of disease" (19–20). He goes on to expound on the impact of fear, joy, hope, anger, jealousy, love, grief, and other "passions." Interestingly, he notes that fear "is a base passion and beneath the dignity of man" (20).

The most important element of this book, however, is the one that my mother used most often, and that was the important inclusion of plant medicine. The value of making sure we understood the use of plants to treat disease and to provide tonics for prevention, and the importance of keeping our emotions in check, pretty much provided us with a willingness to listen to others who made the mind-body-nature connection something real.

In a conversation about getting younger Kituwahs to realize the importance of language and culture and their impact on one's worldview, we spoke of how loss of language and culture or cultural genocide is still a battle being fought every day for Indigenous communities. Tom reminded me that you don't have to kill a person to make them feel dead. Riding this train of thought back to health, he continued that language—that thing that ties you uniquely to your tribal heritage ancestry—is the critical issue. The impact of language loss is pervasive for the individual, community, and nation. Genocide includes the loss of people due to language loss, that loss of identity, which can be an important factor in substance abuse, suicide, and other mental/physical health issues. In my many years working with Native youth and addictions, there were countless comments by patients who "didn't know who they were," were "ashamed of being an Indian," "didn't know how to be an Indian," or "weren't connected to their ceremonies and culture."

Knowing who you are and being connected to place and others are critical in a tribal community and I would also say in a mountain community. Even those who have left Appalachia still refer to the land and community they left, regardless of how many years ago, as their home. That strong identity with place goes with you, and when you return, often it is the family cemetery, church, homeplace, or natural site(s) that you revisit. Ties to family are important. When one works in a community, often the first thing people may ask is "who's your family?" A connection must be made so that you can be placed by lineage and geography. Even being from the northern part of a county or the southern part of a county can be very different in terms of history, family experiences, and perceptions. Historically this location could be instantly detected by one's dialect, which provided a link to family and place. With greater mobility and change, this may no longer be applicable to most of a region. Regardless, connection to people and place is critical in one's identity.

Something as simple as a wave to someone, reflected linguistically in the Kituwah language, possesses a deeper meaning. Tom explains that *gv yo li ha* (ᎬᏲᎵᎰ) means "I am waving at you or greeting you." This comes from the word *gv yo li ga* (ᎬᏲᎵᎦ, I recognize you or I know you), which can mean I know what someone is about. I feel comfortable with you because I understand you and know who you are. I know more than your name, I know what you're about. We are connected in our understanding in how we see the world and its meaning. Our spirituality and purpose are alike.

There is a comfort and sense of peace in knowing that you are a valued member of a family. I watched a Canadian commercial online recently that was simple, yet powerful and moving. There were no words, but the message was clear: we are happier with others. A woman in an apartment building convinced her roommate to put a table and chairs out in the hall with their dinner on it. Pretty soon each of her neighbors came and joined her, sharing their own foods and contributions, making for a joyful meal together; former strangers, now friends. To be included improves our outlook and level of self-worth. For Kituwahs, you can see the instant bonding and camaraderie with others they may not know personally, but both are speaking the language, acknowledging that bond.

In thinking of *tohi* and good well-being, I'm reminded of the words of several elders, not all Cherokees, who wanted me to remember foundational principles from their teachings about good health. One of the most common ones was "the medicine is already within you," which, again, is a lesson from Native science that Western science is acknowledging. Our brains have unlocked secrets of neurochemicals that can fight disease, and that meditation, belief, and the power of psychoneuroimmunology can intervene in.

Michael Yellow Bird (Arikara Nation) has been presenting and writing about decolonizing our minds. He discusses the power of meditation, comparable to the state of mind and body during ceremony, in changing the brain. Delivering the 2018 Annual Public Lecture in Native Health at Western Carolina University, he said that "neuroscience research confirms that mindfulness practices can positively change our brain's structure and function . . . improving awareness and concentration, easing the effects of trauma, raising optimism and fortifying emotional self-regulation, creating a sense of calm, increasing resilience, and reducing conflict."

A "colonized mind" is one that is taught or socialized to break everything down to its smallest element. We aren't often taught how to de-silo disciplines and recognize how things are connected. From a European perspective, we tend to categorize and compartmentalize people, things, areas of study, and beliefs. We want to create hierarchies and see the world in stark black-and-white terms, which makes things "easier" to deal with or ignore. We rarely take the time to see how our actions and beliefs can be connected to multiple issues. For example, we justify cutting down trees and mountains, and polluting the air, soil, and water, or commandeering a glorious view with a trophy house, by just focusing on the monetary value of these various natural resources. There is no real consciousness in that way of thinking. There is no connection to what is living and how it can affect others. Most industrialists who sacrifice these natural resources don't live where they have to experience the toxicity and devastating results of their decisions. That's why, historically, most of the toxic waste dumps, mining, and exploitation of land, water, and air occur on the land of minorities and those historically underserved. Conveniently, their actions of destruction follow a history of colonization. Tom adds, "That's the insidiousness of colonization, is that the colonizers have perpetuated their own perspective of history on those it has most detrimentally impacted, and they just accepted what had been taught to them."

As Tom and I were discussing how difficult it must have been for those Kituwahs who were removed in the early nineteenth century, we spoke in particular about those who were considered leaders, who had to negotiate with white people of the colonizing society about the extraction of their people to the west, a direction that traditionally had symbolized darkness and death. Those leaders, some who promoted leaving their homeland to save lives, some who promoted resistance at all costs, must have been under an incredible burden to do "what was right." Tom used the word *di gu go di sgi* (ᏗᎫᎪᏗᏍᎩ), which means "judge" or "the one who makes things correct." This word comes from *du yu go dv hi*, a variation for the word "judge" that comes from the now-familiar root *du yu go dv i*, "the right way or the right path." The difficulty was that those who had been raised in the Kituwah traditional teachings of making things right in the best possible way for others had to navigate a new world of Europeans whose cultural values of sacredness and spirituality could be compartmentalized. They as colonizers could silo their spiritual values of mercy, kindness, and love, which looked much like those of Kituwahs, and express in their dealings with Indigenous peoples the values of greed, dominion, and accumulation of wealth. Cherokees must have thought us schizophrenic to be able to preach mercy and love while simultaneously dispensing exploitation and horrifying oppression. They saw this as a way of thought that had no life, no conscious. Cherokee historian John R. Finger (1984) wrote, "While the stubborn [Chief] Yonaguska lived, however, the Quallatown Cherokees received little encouragement for adopting the white man's religion. The old chief thought Christian theology embodied some wonderful concepts but, like many Indians before him, noted that Christian doctrine frequently stood in stark contrast to white behavior. Such a religion, he thought, was probably not worth much and was certainly less satisfying than traditional Cherokee ritual and belief" (62).

Even other travelers in Cherokee territory had similar observations. Geologist George William Featherstonhaugh "lamented that the Cherokees were being 'driven from their religious and social state . . .' not because they cannot be civilized, but because a pseudo set of civilized beings, who are too strong for them, want their possessions" (Anderson 1991, 43).

Even many of us who are not Indigenous, who have not faced the same horrific historical trauma, understand this paradox in our society today. It is not that I am trying to throw Christianity under the bus, but the existence of self-identified Christians who can rationalize hate, separation of families, and the destruction of our vital basic elements that we all need for survival is fodder for the cognitive dissonance that dominates our politics, economy, and spiritual conversations. These are the elements of the mind of the colonizers.

Yellow Bird (2018) goes on to explain the "science of colonization," "by invasion, forced entry of your cultural space; manipulation of cultural values, beliefs, and traditions to eradicate them; domination by imposing policies and standards contrary to Indigenous culture; and control of thinking and behavior." The process of colonization is ongoing for Indigenous people, in marginalization, stereotyping, and the imposition of policies and standards of practice that are contrary to those of tribal people.

This occurs in our academies and health-care institutions when cultural values and traditional knowledge are disregarded. By treating all Native people as though they were one monolithic population, we strip them of the rich diversity of their languages and histories and the lessons they contain. We continue to assimilate by creating and mandating standards of "best practice" that may or may not be feasible for some communities. We have an opportunity to listen to tribal people and incorporate the best of both worlds in education and health practice, to value traditional knowledge as a viable way of knowing that can add important lenses with which to examine the problems that affect our communities.

Now is a critical time to support and listen to young Native scholars such as Joseph P. Gone (Gros Ventre), psychologist at Harvard; Clint Carroll (Cherokee), ethnobotanist at the University of Colorado; Trey Adcock (Cherokee), head of Indigenous studies at the University of North Carolina at Asheville; and Cliff and Constance Owl (EBCI). Cliff is a PhD candidate in psychology in California. His sister Constance, at Stanford University, is interested in how interpreting Cherokee historical documents in the language shows a much different and richer perspective of the reality of Cherokee interactions in early Contact. EBCI member Tonya Carrol works for the Tribe in a program with young leaders sharing cultural values and language-based knowledge. Her brother, Bo, is a tribal archaeologist who works closely with elders to aid in better understanding his work. Other siblings from the Cherokee Nation are Melissa and Courtney Lewis. Melissa is at the University of Minnesota, working in health care, and Courtney is at the University of South Carolina, supporting a better understanding of what more "traditional" economics might look like for sovereign nations. Jillian Fish (Tuscarora Nation), Michelle Johnson-Jennings (Choctaw), and Melodi Wynne (Spokane Tribe of Indians) are up-and-coming Native scholars promoting the use of both Native and Western science to address issues of mental health, environmental destruction, climate change, and a host of other social and health issues. They are part of the future of Native communities reaching into the language and the science it holds to make this world a better place.

It takes a concerted effort and a good amount of time to engage Indigenous elders and speakers of their language to develop culturally appropriate models of prevention and intervention for communities. But the time, energy, and effort would be well worth it to develop programs that are finally effective in addressing health disparities and issues of social and environmental justice. The solutions to these problems lie within these communities, not outside. We all strive for peace of mind and well-being. But we will have to "be still" and listen to move forward in humility and value our common ground.

AFTERWORD

Listening to the Sounds of Tohi

This is a book with a message. Looking back only to look forward, this small volume speaks with outsized promise. It arrives as the gift of two deeply humane people, both of the same place in the southern mountains, who came together around the principle that wisdom can and must be shared and that nothing could be lost in the exchange. This takes courage for Cherokees and traditional Appalachian people. Memories of gifts turned into transactions or outright theft have made this kind of dialogue difficult. Like other voices from Indigenous peoples around the world today, this work asserts ethical and spiritual beliefs, rooted in place, in order to pull together worlds that threaten to pull apart. Tom Belt and Lisa Lefler unite perspectives and beliefs that are shared between Cherokee and Appalachian communities.

The connections between their respective communities are, in one sense, geographical. They have lived as mountain neighbors for generations, though living together has not always been easy. The shock of colonization, the intercultural violence of Removal, and two centuries of corrosive dismissal and derision of both Cherokee and Appalachian people and cultures have not made life easy for either group. Together, they speak across a past full of hurt toward a future of shared healing. *Sounds of* Tohi pulls us all together in a world that, in contrast, threatens to pull apart.

This volume arrives at a troubled time for our earthbound human species (though some of us are looking for tickets to Mars). The power behind the words of both communities comes out of the places in the southern Appalachians in which both traditions share their roots. Yet it also offers a message of hope resonant with the many thousands of other worlds and traditions that collectively root life in our globalized "world." *Sounds of* Tohi puts Kituwah religion and kindred Appalachian traditional knowledge standing side by side among the world's living wisdom traditions. It joins with Indigenous voices worldwide, echoing in many languages: "we are still here."

◇◇◇◇◇◇◇◇◇◇◇

Cherokee people maintain a very real memory of how they have struggled, not to take, but to keep their place. As Tom Belt says, being "not from, but of, this place," specifically Kituwah and the mountains around it. In the Kituwah system nothing separates people from the land. "We are the people of the soil that is owned by someone unknown to us." From the perspective of racing modernity and consumerism, place-centered beliefs appear as dusty artifacts of bygone life. However, sacred places do not belong on Zillow. The truth is that place-connected communities live on into the present in their place. Our species is wired for attachment with place and homeland. The degree to which this instinct can be perverted into territorial allegiance and flag-carrying aggressions is simply a superficial reflection of its depth. Despite their late arrival in the neighborhood, Appalachian settlers and their descendants learned from their elders, but also directly felt the soul-bending life force of the oldest mountains of the world.

As Edwin Bernbaum's book *Sacred Mountains of the World* (1990) showed more than thirty years ago, there is a globalized tendency to look up to the peaks for understanding. This holds true from Denali, to Kilimanjaro, to Sagarmatha, the star seeker of the Himalayas, to the Minoan sanctuary at Mount Juktas, overlooking Heraklion. Pilgrims still seek thousands of such places. Of course, mountains are markers of something much larger, as this book makes clear. Standing on the ground at Kituwah, or on the campus of Western Carolina University, which occupies a deeply important Cherokee traditional place, we find connections in both sky and body. And there are personal connections as well. Connections that led to this book.

And it is, of course, not just the peaks, but the entire connective tissue of valley, river, foothills, settlement and long-stewarded forest that surrounds them. This pattern underlies at ground level the cosmographic maps connected to Cherokee heroes like Judaculla, the giant. The campus of Western Carolina University is located in Cullowhee, occupying a shallow soup bowl of a valley, at the center of a deeply important spiritual landscape. The Cherokee name of this ancient place is Judaculla's place, and Judaculla's story creates cosmography by linking Judaculla's rock, the steep balsam drainages to the east, "Devil's Courthouse" (as Judaculla's seat came to be derisively known to settlers fearful of pagan beliefs) and "Waterrock Knob" to the west, and outward in other directions. It is not hard to see how so much within *Sounds of* Tohi emerges at least in part from Judaculla's place and other ever-expanding dialogues, such as Rooted in the Mountains, which Lisa and Tom created.

A metes and bounds survey might measure Judaculla's domain as encompassing more than a hundred square miles, but there are manifold dimensions here. In fact, the cosmography has nothing to do with measurement. T. J. Holland's painting on the book's cover portrays with great beauty the "petroglyphs" left by Judaculla on his "rock" along the Caney Fork River on the turned head of an observer. The figure in the portrait looks out toward the horizon in a reflection of internalized unity between person, place, and cosmos. It is a visual expression of the spiritual lines mapped on Judaculla Rock and the sky, but also embodied in the Kituwah believer. The broader dimensions of what it means for the university and the region to occupy "Judaculla's place" are just beginning to emerge.

◇◇◇◇◇◇◇◇◇◇◇

In more than ten thousand or fifteen thousand years of living in the deep valleys of the mountain landscape, Cherokee ancestors responded cyclically to sudden episodes of environmental, climatic, and social change. This deep knowledge provides new tools to navigate complex challenges ahead. Appalachian traditional science can enrich concepts such as resilience, risk, and sustainability in how to reduce uncertainty in navigating toward a broader collective health. The importance of this is emerging.

It is possibly not an accident that this book follows the "right path" during global distress wrought by a simple virus. A simple virus carried by the bats or the humble scaled mammal, the pangolin, or creatures unknown illustrates how all parts of life and all spaces of life are interconnected—negatively or positively. If the lives and the habitats of pangolins and bats had been respected, and if inherently placeless megacities were built from a blueprint of health rather than consumption, perhaps we could have avoided or at least better absorbed this shock. As *Sounds of* Tohi makes clear, there is no real "human-animal" barrier that we must reinforce. Rather, we need to embrace and accommodate our relatedness.

International law, often seen as the bastard child of capitalism, can do more. It can find a fulcrum for overriding the dependence of small people on the sanction and approbation of nation-states. Local connects to global. Without the survival of the small-world traditions, languages, and systems of knowledge, we all lose an anchoring stability.

◇◇◇◇◇◇◇◇◇◇◇

This book is a singularly generous act of following *duyuk'dv'i*, the right path. Motivated by a sense of the right time, not just for the authors but also for the future of their communities, it offers guideposts for at-risk Cherokee and people of place around the world who have remained quiet so as to survive. It is a response to a deepening crisis in their communities, a message to a new generation, as well as to other peoples. It is also an offer of healing wisdom shared as a gift that incurs no loss to the giver. In this, it responds to the fact that today the traumas of small places, noticed or not by global news, are ultimately amplified on a global scale.

Most of all, *Sounds of* Tohi is an offer of what Rabbi Jonathan Sacks in *To Heal a Fractured World* (2005) calls the "ethics of responsibility." Repeated in daily prayer in the synagogue, the Hebrew phrase *tikkun olam* metaphorically reflects how our "acts make a difference." Our acts can "repair old fractures in the world. They restore a lost order. They rescue fragments of divine light" (78). The Kituwah way, and its ethical precepts of *tohi*, *duyuk'dv'i*, and others, offers an equally compelling message of conduct and responsibility much like *tikkun olam*, concerned with order. The book provides a glimpse at this foundation of what this ordering might look like in a reinvention of our nation.

A new collective polity is possible with acknowledgment, full inclusion, and in all senses *recognition* of the nearly five hundred tribal nations in the United States. The profound but urgent humilities of the Kituwah and Appalachian people provide a civic vision not just for the Cherokee people. A founding Puritan myth was that the American nation was destined to become a "city upon a hill." *Sounds of* Tohi should remind us all of the necessity of building a more equitable nation, rooted in many ancient places, and honoring their inhabitants. It reminds us of how our collective futures depend on how we care, not just for the city, but for the hill itself.

TOM HATLEY
ASHEVILLE, NC

ACKNOWLEDGMENTS

All writers, of fiction and nonfiction, are able to process and tell their stories with the help of others. Our stories are shared and created by the experiences we live and learn from others. We are social animals who need others to learn about love, hope, overcoming, and the lessons in life that make us who we are. And for many of us, those "others" may also include the life that comes in the form of animals and the natural world around us, as many Indigenous peoples say, "all our relations."

I cannot begin to note all the people through the many years that have taught me lessons of living and even the prospect of dying. Trauma and the short-sightedness of youth prevented me from mining the hard questions from elders about wisdom and ancestry, and about how things have come to be. I don't want to fail my friends and relatives by not acknowledging how the intersection of our lives has forever affected me. I am humbled by both my many mistakes in life and my successes. I know that the more I know, I know that I don't really know, but I'm still willing to learn. An anthropologist that I admired early in my career said that the formula for wisdom is wonder, always remaining curious, and humility, the ability to shut up and listen for as long as it takes to learn. Good advice I continue to value today.

I want to make sure to note the contributions of Pam, TJ, and both Toms included in this volume. They are family. They make me laugh, think, and feel loved, and I love them. I learn from them all the time and am so grateful for their friendship and trust. I also thank their families, Roseanna Belt, Caroline Holland, Jane Hatley, and Kelly Duncan for their patience as this book interrupted their lives. Y'all have the patience of Job. We appreciate the expertise and help of Ben Jensen in translation to the Cherokee syllabary. Thank you to my dear friends Vickie Bradley (Eastern Band of Cherokee Indians), secretary of health for the EBCI, and Rosemary Peek, who never failed to offer their services in feedback and editing throughout this process. Rosemary also provided the photos. I'm grateful for the time and energy of Katsi

Cook (Mohawk) who has been kind enough to allow me in her community and who traveled here to Cherokee homeland to teach and help us in our work. I also want to thank Charles Radcliffe for his help in formatting and working to get this manuscript ready, Jessica Hinds-Bond for her diligence in editing and indexing, and Wendi Schnaufer at the University of Alabama Press for her hard work in shepherding this manuscript through the process. I also want to acknowledge the work and contributions to the understanding and application of traditional ecological knowledge (TEK) from my friends and colleagues of the Smithsonian Health and Culture Work Group. Thanks to Wendell Berry and his daughter, Mary, for allowing us the privilege of reprinting his work, which I have admired for so many years. Thanks as well to Jackson County Library for space for Tom and I to record our talks, to City Lights Bookstore for a quiet place to read and meet others, to the many Cherokee and other tribal elders who shared their experiences and time, and to my furry children, who provided some much-needed dog therapy. Thanks to Newfound Press at the University of Tennessee for permission to use in chapter 3 material previously published in Lisa J. Lefler, "Traditional Knowledge and Health: Lessons from the Eastern Band of Cherokee Indians," in *Anthropology: Weaving Our Discipline with Community*, edited by Lisa J. Lefler (Knoxville, TN: Newfound Press, 2020), 109–26.

I am continually amazed at how important humor is in aiding resiliency and fertilizing grounds for kindness, trust, respect, and even love for one another. Working among Appalachian and Native peoples provides that in spades. Thanks to *all my relations* for making the stories, music, food, and understanding about the land and cultures in which we live joyful, healing, and meaningful, not just for those of us who live in Appalachia, but for people everywhere there is connection to place.

LISA J. LEFLER
DILLSBORO, NORTH CAROLINA

FURTHER READING

On Alternative Genders and Native Americans

Brown, Lester B., ed. 1997. *Two Spirit People: American Indian Lesbian Women and Gay Men*. New York: Haworth Press.

Gilley, Brian Joseph. 2006. *Becoming Two-Spirit: Gay Identity and Social Acceptance in Indian Country*. Lincoln: University of Nebraska Press.

Herdt, Gilbert, ed. 1993. *Third Sex, Third Gender: Beyond Sexual Dimorphism in Culture and History*. New York: Zone Books.

Jacobs, Sue-Ellen, Wesley Thomas, and Sabine Lang, eds. 1997. *Two Spirit People: Native American Gender Identity, Sexuality, and Spirituality*. Chicago: University of Illinois Press.

Lang, Sabine. 1998. *Men as Women, Women as Men: Changing Gender in Native American Cultures*. Austin: University of Texas Press.

Roscoe, Will. 1991. *The Zuni Man-Woman*. Albuquerque: University of New Mexico Press.

———. 1998. *Changing Ones: Third and Fourth Genders in Native North America*. New York: St. Martin's Press.

William, Walter L. 1986. *The Spirit and the Flesh: Sexual Diversity in American Indian Culture*. Boston: Beacon Press.

On Cherokee Women

Carney, Virginia Moore. 2005. *Eastern Band Cherokee Women: Cultural Persistence in Their Letters and Speeches*. Knoxville: University of Tennessee Press.

Hill, Sarah H. 1997. *Weaving New Worlds: Southeastern Cherokee Women and Their Basketry*. Chapel Hill: University of North Carolina Press.

Johnston, Carolyn. 2003. *Cherokee Women in Crisis: Trail of Tears, Civil War, and Allotment, 1838–1907*. Tuscaloosa: University of Alabama Press.

Purdue, Theda. 1998. *Cherokee Women: Gender and Culture Change, 1700–1835*. Lincoln: University of Nebraska Press.

Traditional Histories and Ethnographies

Finger, John R. 1984. *The Eastern Band of Cherokees, 1819–1900*. Knoxville: University of Tennessee Press.

———. 1991. *Cherokee Americans: The Eastern Band of Cherokees in the Twentieth Century.* Lincoln: University of Nebraska Press.

Gilbert, William H. 1943. *The Eastern Cherokees.* Washington, DC: Smithsonian Institution Bureau of Ethnology.

McLoughlin, William G. 1986. *Cherokee Renascence in the New Republic.* Princeton, NJ: Princeton University Press.

Mooney, James. (1891–1900) 1982. *History, Myths, and Sacred Formulas of the Cherokees.* Nashville, TN: Charles and Randy Elder Booksellers.

Neely, Sharlotte. 1991. *Snowbird Cherokees: People of Persistence.* Athens: University of Georgia Press.

REFERENCES

Albrecht, Glenn. 2010. "Solastalgia and the Creation of New Ways of Living." In *Nature and Culture: Rebuilding Lost Connections*, edited by Sarah Pilgrim and Jules N. Pretty, 217–34. London: Routledge.

Altman, Heidi M., and Thomas N. Belt. 2009. "*Tohi*: The Cherokee Concept of Well-Being." In *Under the Rattlesnake: Cherokee Health and Resiliency*, edited by Lisa J. Lefler, 9–22. Tuscaloosa: University of Alabama Press.

Anderson, Gary Clayton. 2014. *Ethnic Cleansing and the Indian*. Norman: University of Oklahoma Press.

Anderson, William L., ed. 1991. *Cherokee Removal*. Athens: University of Georgia Press.

Ballard, E. D., K. Van Eck, R. J. Musci, S. R. Hart, C. L. Storr, N. Breslau, and H. C. Wilcox. 2015. "Latent Classes of Childhood Trauma Exposure Predict the Development of Behavioral Health Outcomes in Adolescence and Young Adulthood." *Psychological Medicine* 45 (15): 3305–16.

Bartels, Meghan. 2019. "NASA and Navajo Nation Partner in Understanding the Universe." Space.com. February 25, 2019. https://www.space.com.

Belt, Thomas N. 2019. "An Introduction to Where We Are: Giduwagi." Keynote address, Rooted in the Mountains Annual Symposium, Western Carolina University, Cullowhee, NC, September 26, 2019.

Berkhofer, Robert. 1965. *Salvation and the Savage: An Analysis of Protestant Missions and American Indian Response, 1787–1862*. Lexington: University of Kentucky Press.

Bernbaum, Edwin. 1990. *Sacred Mountains of the World*. Berkeley: University of California Press.

Berry, Wendell. 1995. *Another Turn of the Crank*. Berkeley, CA: Counterpoint Press.

———. 2002. *The Art of the Commonplace*. Berkeley, CA: Counterpoint Press.

———. 2018. *The Peace of Wild Things*. London: Penguin Random House.

Cajete, Gregory. 2004. "Philosophy of Native Science." In *American Indian Thought*, edited by Anne Waters, 45–57. Malden, MA: Blackwell.

Cheng, Wei-Wen, Chien-Tsong Lin, Fang-Hua Chu, Shang-Tzen Chang, and

Sheng-Yang Wang. 2009. "Neuropharmacological Activities of Phytoncide Released from *Cryptomeria japonica.*" *Journal of Wood Science* 55:27–31.

Cook, Katsi. 2012. "Women, Health and Culture." Keynote address, Rooted in the Mountains Annual Symposium, Western Carolina University, Cullowhee, NC, October 4, 2012.

———. 2018. "Woman as the First Environment." Keynote address, Rooted in the Mountains Annual Symposium, Western Carolina University, Cullowhee, NC, September 27, 2018.

Cory, Jessica. 2019. *Mountains Piled upon Mountains: Appalachian Nature Writing in the Anthropocene.* Morgantown: West Virginia University Press.

Crossland, Christine, Jane Palmer, and Alison Brooks. 2013. "NIJ's Program of Research on Violence against American Indian and Alaska Native Women." *Violence against Women* 19 (6): 771–90.

Cumfer, Cynthia. 2007. *Separate Peoples, One Land: The Minds of Cherokees, Blacks, and Whites on the Tennessee Frontier.* Chapel Hill: University of North Carolina Press.

Deloria, Vine, Jr. 1979. *Metaphysics of Modern Existence.* New York: Harper and Row.

Driskill, Qwo-Li. 2008. "Shaking Our Shells: Cherokee Two-Spirits Rebalancing the World." In *Beyond Masculinity: Essays by Queer Men on Gender & Politics,* edited by Trevor Hoppe, 121–41. http://www.beyondmasculinity.com.

Duncan, Pamela Y. 2019. "Where I Belong: Mountain Homeplace in Appalachia." Paper presented at Mediating Mountains, the International Conference of the Austrian Association for American Studies, University of Innsbruck, Austria, November 23, 2019.

Duran, Eduardo. 2004. "Intergenerational Trauma." Keynote address, Appalachian Studies Conference, Cherokee, NC.

Erdrich, Louise. 1985. "Where I Ought to Be: A Writer's Sense of Place." *New York Times,* July 28, 1985.

Executive Office of the President (EOP). 2014. *2014 Native Youth Report.* Washington, DC: EOP. https://obamawhitehouse.archives.gov/.

Fedoroff, Nina V. 2003. "Agriculture: Prehistoric GM Corn." *Science* 302 (November 14): 1158–59.

Finger, John R. 1984. *The Eastern Band of Cherokee Indians, 1819–1900.* Knoxville: University of Tennessee Press.

———. 1991. *Cherokee Americans: The Eastern Band of Cherokees in the Twentieth Century.* Lincoln: University of Nebraska Press.

Fogelson, Raymond D. 1977. "Cherokee Notions of Power." In *The Anthropology of Power,* edited by Raymond D. Fogelson and Richard N. Adams, 185–93. New York: Academic Press.

George, Dan, and Helmut Hirnschall. 2003. *The Best of Chief Dan George.* Surrey, BC: Hancock House.

Gilley, Brian Joseph. 2006. *Becoming Two-Spirit: Gay Identity and Social Acceptance in Indian Country.* Lincoln: University of Nebraska Press.

Gone, Joseph P. 2004. "Keeping Culture in Mind: Transforming Academic Training in Professional Psychology for Indian Country." In *Indigenizing the Academy: Transforming Scholarship and Empowering Communities*, edited by D. A. Mihesuah and A. Cavender Wilson, 124–42. Lincoln: University of Nebraska Press.

———. 2017. "Recovering Indigenous Knowledge Traditions for Rethinking Mental Health." Keynote address, Rooted in the Mountains Annual Symposium Western Carolina University, Cullowhee, NC, September 28, 2017.

Gulick, John. 1960. *Cherokees at the Crossroads*. Chapel Hill: Institute for Research in Social Science, University of North Carolina.

Gunn, John C. (1830) 1986. *Gunn's Domestic Medicine*. Knoxville: University of Tennessee Press.

Hari, Johann. 2016. "The Opposite of Addiction Isn't Sobriety—It's Connection." *Guardian*, April 12, 2016.

Harkins, Anthony, and Meredith McCarroll, eds. 2019. *Appalachian Reckoning: A Region Responds to Hillbilly Elegy*. Morgantown: West Virginia University Press.

Hatley, Thomas M. 1995. *The Dividing Paths*. New York: Oxford University Press.

Henri, Florette. 1986. *The Southern Indians and Benjamin Hawkins, 1796–1816*. Norman: University of Oklahoma Press.

Herdt, Gilbert, ed. 1993. *Third Sex, Third Gender: Beyond Sexual Dimorphism in Culture and History*. New York: Zone Books.

House, Silas. 2010. "Thin Places." Keynote address, Rooted in the Mountains Annual Symposium, Western Carolina University, Cullowhee, NC, October 21, 2010.

Howard, Albert. (1995) 2006. *The Soil and Health: A Study of Organic Agriculture*. Lexington: University Press of Kentucky.

Ibrahim, Mohab. 2019. "Researchers Explore a Drug-Free Idea to Relieve Chronic Pain: Green Light." *Morning Edition*. NPR, December 15, 2019. https://www.npr.org.

Jacobs, Sue-Ellen, Wesley Thomas, and Sabine Lang, eds. 1997. *Two Spirit People: Native American Gender Identity, Sexuality, and Spirituality*. Chicago: University of Illinois Press.

James, Jenny. 2009. "Sacred Feminine in Cherokee Culture." In *Under the Rattlesnake: Cherokee Health and Resiliency*, edited by Lisa J. Lefler, 102–24. Tuscaloosa: University of Alabama Press.

Johnson, Greg. 2011. Untitled presentation. "Religious Freedom, Sacred Sites, and Land Rights" panel. Indigenous Land Rights and Religious Freedom Symposium, Wake Forest University, Winston-Salem, NC, April 7, 2011.

Johnson, S. B., A. W. Riley, D. A. Granger, and J. Riis. 2013. "The Science of Early Life Toxic Stress for Pediatric Practice and Advocacy." *Pediatrics* 131 (2): 319–27.

Jones, David S. 2004. *Rationalizing Epidemics*. Cambridge, MA: Harvard University Press.

Junger, Sebastian. 2016. *Tribe: On Homecoming and Belonging*. New York: Twelve Hatchet Book Group.

King, Charles. 2019. *Gods of the Upper Air: How a Circle of Renegade Anthropologists Reinvented Race, Sex, and Gender in the Twentieth Century*. New York: Doubleday.

Lang, Sabine. 1998. *Men as Women, Women as Men: Changing Gender in Native American Cultures*. Austin: University of Texas Press.

Las Casas, Bartolomé de. (1550) 1992. *In Defense of the Indians*. Translated by C. M. Stafford Poole. DeKalb: Northern Illinois University Press.

Lefler, Hugh Talmage, and Albert Ray Newsome. 1954. *North Carolina: The History of a Southern State*. Chapel Hill: University of North Carolina Press.

Lefler, Lisa J., ed. 2009. *Under the Rattlesnake: Cherokee Health and Resiliency*. Tuscaloosa: University of Alabama Press.

———. 2020. "Traditional Knowledge and Health: Lessons from the Eastern Band of Cherokee Indians." In *Anthropology: Weaving Our Discipline with Community*, edited by Lisa J. Lefler, 109–26. Knoxville, TN: Newfound Press.

Makepeace, Anne, dir. 2010. *We Still Live Here*. Oley, PA: Bullfrog Films. DVD, 56 min.

Malone, Henry T. 1957. "Cherokee-White Relations on the Southern Frontier in the Early Nineteenth Century." *North Carolina Historical Review* 34 (1): 1–14.

Manning, Maurice. 2006. "Maurice Manning on Verlyn Klinkenborg's *Timothy; or, Notes of an Abject Reptile*." *BookForum*, February/March 2006.

Martin-Hill, Dawn. 2008. *The Lubicon Lake Nation: Indigenous Knowledge and Power*. Toronto: University of Toronto Press.

McCarroll, Meredith. 2018. *Un-White: Appalachia, Race, and Film*. Athens: University of Georgia Press.

McDowell, William L., ed. 1958. *Documents Relating to Indian Affairs, 1750–1754*. Vol. 1. Columbia: South Carolina Department of Archives and History.

McLoughlin, William G. 1986. *Cherokee Renascence in the New Republic*. Princeton, NJ: Princeton University Press.

Momaday, N. Scott. 1988. "Sacred and Ancestral Ground." *New York Times*, March 13, 1988.

Montrose, Louis. 1993. "The Work of Gender in the Discourse of Discovery." In *New World Encounters*, edited by Stephen Greenblatt, 177–216. Berkeley: University of California Press.

Mooney, James. (1891–1900) 1982. *History, Myths, and Sacred Formulas of the Cherokees*. Nashville, TN: Charles and Randy Elder Booksellers.

National Institute on Alcohol Abuse and Alcoholism (NIAAA). 2020. "Substance Abuse Prevention for Youth in Indigenous Communities." Webinar. October 8, 2020. https://www.niaaa.nih.gov.

Neely, Sharlotte. 1991. *Snowbird Cherokees: People of Persistence*. Athens: University of Georgia Press.

Olson, Lenora, and Stephanie Wahab. 2006. "American Indians and Suicide: A Neglected Area of Research." *Trauma, Violence, and Abuse* 7 (1): 19–33.

Oxford University Press. n.d. Lexico.com. Accessed December 1, 2021. https://www.lexico.com.

Peat, F. David. 2002. *Blackfoot Physics: A Journey into the Native American World-view.* Boston: Weiser Books.

Perdue, Charles L., Jr., and Nancy J. Martin-Perdue. 1979–80. "Appalachian Fables and Facts: A Case Study of the Shenandoah National Park Removals." *Appalachian Journal* 7 (1/2): 84–104.

Prucha, Francis Paul. 1984. *The Great Father: The United States Government and the American Indians.* Lincoln: University of Nebraska Press.

Reece, Chuck. 2020. "Hillbillies Need No Elegy." *The Bitter Southerner.* Podcast. February 7, 2020. https://bittersoutherner.com.

Riggs, Brett H. 1999. "Removal Period Cherokee Households in Southwestern North Carolina: Material Perspectives on Ethnicity and Cultural Differentiation." PhD diss., University of Tennessee, Knoxville.

Roscoe, Will. 1991. *The Zuni Man-Woman.* Albuquerque: University of New Mexico Press.

———. 1998. *Changing Ones: Third and Fourth Genders in Native North America.* New York: St. Martin's Press.

Sacks, Jonathan. 2005. *To Heal a Fractured World.* New York: Schocken Books.

Selhub, Eva. 2021. "A Doctor Explains How to Take Advantage of the Healing Powers of Nature." Mind Body Green. Last updated February 23, 2021. https://www.mindbodygreen.com.

Smith, Herb, dir. 1984. *Strangers and Kin: A History of the Hillbilly Image.* Whitesburg, KY: Appalshop. Film, 59 min.

Smithers, Gregory D. 2014. "Cherokee 'Two Spirits': Gender, Ritual, and Spirituality in the Native South." *Early American Studies* 12 (3): 626–51.

———. 2015. *The Cherokee Diaspora: An Indigenous History of Migration, Resettlement, and Identity.* New Haven, CT: Yale University Press.

Sohn, Pam. 2009. "Cherokees Mark Historic Gathering at Red Clay." *Chattanooga Times Free Press,* April 17, 2009.

Stannard, David E. 1992a. *American Holocaust: The Conquest of the New World.* New York: Oxford University Press.

———. 1992b. "Genocide in the Americas." *Nation,* October 19, 1992.

Tannen, Deborah. 2007. *You Just Don't Understand: Women and Men in Conversation.* New York: HarperCollins.

Taylor, Jill Bolte. 2008. "A Brain Scientist with a 'Stroke of Insight.'" Interview. *Fresh Air.* NPR, June 25, 2008. https://www.npr.org.

———. 2009. *My Stroke of Insight: A Brain Scientist's Personal Journey.* New York: Plume.

Thomas, Robert K. 1958. "Cherokee Values and World View." Unpublished manuscript, University of North Carolina, Chapel Hill.

Timberlake, Henry. (1765) 1948. *Lieut. Henry Timberlake's Memoirs, 1756–1765.* Marietta, GA: Samuel Cole Williams.

Timberlake Scholarly Symposium. 2006. Museum of the Cherokee Indian, Cherokee, NC, April 25, 2006.

Trafzer, Clifford E., and Joel R. Hyer, eds. 1999. *Exterminate Them! Written*

Accounts of the Murder, Rape, and Enslavement of Native Americans during the California Gold Rush. East Lansing: Michigan State University Press.

Vance, J. D. 2016. *Hillbilly Elegy: A Memoir of a Family and Culture in Crisis*. New York: HarperCollins.

Veteto, James, Gary Paul Nabhan, Regina Fitzsimmons, Kanin Routson, and Deja Walker, eds. 2011. *Place-Based Foods of Appalachia: From Rarity to Community Restoration and Market Recovery*. https://garynabhan.com.

Wahrhaftig, Albert L. 1970. *Social and Economic Characteristics of the Cherokee Population of Eastern Oklahoma: Report of a Survey of Four Cherokee Settlements in the Cherokee Nation*. Washington, DC: American Anthropological Association.

Werito, Vincent. 2014. "Understanding *Hozho* to Achieve Critical Consciousness: A Contemporary Diné Interpretation of the Philosophical Principles of *Hozho*." In *Diné Perspectives: Revitalizing and Reclaiming Navajo Thought*, edited by Lloyd L. Lee, 25–38. Tucson: University of Arizona Press.

Western Carolina University. n.d. "Two Sparrows Town: The Ancient Cherokee Community Emerges Again." Accessed October 1, 2021. https://www.wcu.edu/.

Williams, Walter L. 1986. *The Spirit and the Flesh: Sexual Diversity in American Indian Culture*. Boston: Beacon Press.

Wood, Peter H. 1992. "When Old Worlds Meet." *Southern Exposure* 20 (1): 14–45.

Wunder, John R. 2000. "'Merciless Indian Savages' and the Declaration of Independence: Native Americans Translate the Ecunnaunuxulgee Document." *American Indian Law Review* 25 (1): 65–92.

Yellow Bird, Michael. 2018. "Neurodecolonization and Indigenous Mindfulness." Annual Public Lecture in Native Health, Western Carolina University, Cullowhee, NC, September 5, 2018.

INDEX

Page numbers in *italics* indicate figures.

Aboriginal Dreamtime, 70
ada ge yu di (to hold on to one another), 75
a da na te di (thought), 60, 76
a da na to gi (heart), 60, 76
Adcock, Trey, 80
addiction. *See* substance abuse
a di tas go i (alcoholism), 13
adverse childhood experience (ACE) scores, 58
Alaska Native populations, 2, 19–20, 55
Albrecht, Glenn, 36
alcoholism, xvi, 2, 13–15, 22, 45, 56. *See also* substance abuse
Alexander, Bruce, 54
alternative gendered people, 19–20
Altman, Heidi M., 12–13
Amazons, 24
American Dream, 37
Anderson, Gary Clayton, 65
Anderson, William, 25
Anglo-Cherokee War, 25
aniKituwah (one town), 50
anxiety, 55
Appalachian people: and managing emotions, 74, 76; negative stereotypes about, xiii–xiv, 2–3; published histories of, 8–9; and rootedness of, xi–xii, xiv–xxi, 7, 34, 77, 82–83; and "thin places," 40–41

Appalachian Studies Association, xiv, 40
Appalshop, xiv
Arikara Nation, 78
asga e ha (harm), 73
assimilation, 21, 23, 44, 53–54, 66, 69, 76, 80
a tse i (the color green), 64

Baird, Jesse Little Doe, 37
Bass, Tommie, 35
Battiste, Marie, 31
Battle of Little Big Horn, 72
Begay, David, 33
Belt, Tom: on the "beginning place," 71–72; on ceremony, 12, 14–15, 60, 67–68, 74–75; on Cherokee language, 3, 5, 10–12, 18, 50, 53, 64, 73–74, 77; on colonialism/meanness, 25, 65–66, 78–79; on connection to place, xxi, 16–17, 41–45, 49, 64, 83; on horses, 68–69; on Kituwah name, 16–17, 44, 72; on Kituwah way, 47–48, 73–76; and Jean Lefler, ix–x, xvii–xviii, 12, 64; life/family of, xi, xiv, xx–xxi, 45, 47–48, 68, 75; on natural laws, 59, 69; on "two hearts," 19
berdache (two spirits), 19–20
Berkhofer, Robert, 65
Bernbaum, Edwin, 83

Berry, Wendell, xix, 1, 34
Bitter Southerner, The (podcast), xiv
Blackfoot, 33, 68
Blue Ridge Parkway, xiv
Boas, Franz, 1
Bohm, David, 6–7
botanical medicine, xv–xvi, 15, 29–30, 34–35, 76
Boundary, the, 52
Brooks, Alison, 20
Brown, Lester B., 19

Cajete, Gregory, 30
Canada, 77
Caney Fork, North Carolina, xix, 41
Caney Fork River, 84
Carrol, Bo, 80
Carrol, Tonya, 80
Carroll, Clint, 80
Center for Cherokee Plants, 30
Center for Native Health, 32–33
ceremony: and healing, 12, 14–15, 51, 78; and Kituwah identity, 37, 48–49, 58, 74–75; as reminder of what is true, 60–61, 67–68, 70. *See also* traditional knowledge
Cherokee, North Carolina, xx–xxi, 16–17, 35, 44–45, 83
Cherokee language: on colonialism, 65–66; and counseling, 6, 61; as identity, 52–53, 58, 71, 74; as medicine, 10–12, 35, 50, 75; and "old way of knowing," 46–47, 64–65; and the sacred, 3–5, 11–12, 35; spatial orientation of, xi, xvii–xviii, 44; on stress/fear, 73; syllabary/sounds of, 4, 13, 21, 64; youth and, 52–53, 76–77
Cherokee Lower Towns, 22
Cherokee Middle Towns, 25
Cherokee Nation, 16, 23, 51, 80
Cherokee people: botanical knowledge of, 29–30, 38; clan system, 21, 25–27, 69, 77; creation story of, 17, 26–27, 44; cultural transformation and, 21;

early/published histories of, 8–9, 20, 21–22, 24, 30, 65, 79; and harmony ethic/Kituwah way, 21, 37, 47–49, 70, 74–76; "official" tribes of, 16, 23; resilience of, 22–24, 46, 51, 82, 84; three major laws of, 75; youth, 6, 42–43, 51–53, 55–59, 61–62, 76–77. *See also* cosmography; Eastern Band of Cherokee Indians (ECBI); Indigenous epistemologies; traditional knowledge
Cherokee Removal, xiv, xx–xxi, 22–24, 27, 47, 69, 79, 82
Cherokee Valley Towns, 25
Cherokee women: and community healing, 5, 19–20, 27–28; as life giving, 17–18, *18*, 27, 33; at time of Contact, 5, 24–27; violence against, 20–21, 27–28; and war, 20, 24, 27
Cheyenne, 72
Chickamauga, 25
Choctaw, 80
"city upon a hill," 85
Civil War, xiii
Claxton, Mae, 7
climate change, xiv, 7, 29, 54, 80, 84
colonization: and genocide, 25, 65–66, 77, 79; and loss of identity, 61, 69, 73, 78–80, 82; and women/gender roles, 5, 19–23, 25–26, 28
connectedness: versus addiction, 53–54; and being *of* a place, xii, xvi–xxi, 5, 11–12, 36–37, 44–45, 50–52, 77; generational, xiv–xv, xx–xxi, 51–53, 77; and "green spaces," 63–64; and healing, ix, 10–11, 36–38, 43, 45, 55; and Indigenous epistemologies, 6, 30–33, 37–38, 43–44; and language, 3–5; multiple dimensions of, 46–47, 59, 63, 65, 68–69, 84; of sciences, 6–7; and "thin places," 40–43, 49, 83–84; and three Kituwah laws, 75; urgent need for, 7, 84–85. *See also* Indigenous epistemologies; mountains; traditional knowledge; tribalism

Contact: atrocities of, 65–66, 79; and Cherokee women/gender roles, 5, 19–22, 24–27; and Indigenous epistemologies, 6, 29–30, 69, 80. *See also* colonization

Cook, Katsi, 20, 38, 68

Cory, Jessica, 7

cosmography: and the "beginning place," 71–72; Cherokee creation story, 17, 26–27, 44; Cherokee youth and, 42–43, 51–53, 61; introduced, 6, 39; and Judaculla Rock, 41, *42*; and spirituality, 66–70; "thin places," 40–43, 49, 83–84. *See also* connectedness; "natural laws"

counseling: and Native treatment centers, 55–57, 61–62; and "soul wound" model, 35–36; and traditional knowledge, 2, 6, 14, 43–44, 46, 58–62. *See also* substance abuse; trauma

COVID-19, 66, 84

Cowee Mound, 49

Creek, *18*, 24–25

Crossland, Christine, 20

Crow, 69

Cullowhee, North Carolina, 41, 83

Cumfer, Cynthia, 25–26

Custer, Armstrong, 72

Dakota, 33

Declaration of Independence, 65

decolonizing efforts. *See* colonization; Indigenizing/decolonizing efforts

dehigeyusesdi (you love them), 75

Deloria, Vine, Jr., 6, 30–32

Denali, 83

depression, 36, 44–45, 51, 55, 59

Devil's Courthouse, 41, 83

diabetes, 13–14, 58

di gu go di sgi (judge), 79

di ka nv wa dv sdi (law), 50

Diné, 33, 66, 70

Dragging Canoe, 25

Dreamtime, 70

Driskill, Qwo-Li, 20

Duncan, Pamela Y., 41

Duran, Eduardo, 14, 27, 35–36, 43, 57, 61

duyukʼdvʼi/duyugodvi (the right path): and language as medicine, 3, 11–13, 75; and "natural laws," 5, 45–46, 48–49, 59, 69, 72; and responsible conduct, 79, 84–85; in woodpecker gorget, 17, *18*. See also *tohi* (health)

Eastern Band of Cherokee Indians (EBCI), xx, 16, 23, 27, 30, 39, 41, 52, 73, 80

ela na gi' (everywhere/beginning place), 71–72

Elizabeth, Queen, 24

elo ni gv (paradise), 71, 74

epigenetics, 14, 57

epistemology. *See* Indigenous epistemologies; traditional knowledge; Western epistemologies

Erdrich, Louise, ix

esga uyelvha (depression), 45

ethics of responsibility, 85

Featherstonhaugh, George William, 79

federal recognition status, 23

federal relocation program (1950s), 44

federal youth treatment centers, 55–57, 61–62

Finger, John R., 23, 79

Fish, Jillian, 80

Fogelman, Eva, 14

Fogelson, Raymond D., 26–27

"forest bathing," 64

Fort Armistead, Tennessee, xx

gadugi (making oneself available to serve others), 14, 75

ga lv quo di (to care about one another), 75

genocide, 25, 65–66, 77, 79

George, Chief Dan, 65

Gilley, Brian Joseph, 19

Gods of the Upper Air (King), 1–2

go hi ti (belief), 67

Gone, Joseph P., 14, 43, 53, 58, 60, 61, 80

Grant, James, 49

Great Smoky Mountains, xiv

Greene, Nathan, 25

"green spaces," 63–64

Gros Ventre, 53, 80

Gulick, John, 27

Gunn, John, 76

Gunn's Domestic Medicine, 15, 76

gv yo li ha (I am waving at you), 77

gvyuga (offense), 45

Hales, Hannah, 24

Hari, Johann, 54

Harkins, Anthony, xiv

harmony ethic, 21, 37, 47–49, 70, 74–76

Harvard Brain Tissue Resource Center, 37

Hatley, Thomas M., 22

Hawkins, Benjamin, 24–25

health. See *tohi* (health)

health disparity gaps, 55

Hebrew, 85

Henderson, James, 31

Henri, Florette, 25

Herdt, Gilbert, 19

Hillbilly Elegy (Vance), xiv

Himalayas, 83

Hoffman, Dustin, 65

Holland, T. J., 39, 44, 84

Hopi, 36–37

House, Silas, 40

Howard, Albert, 34

hozho (Diné concept of harmony), 70

Hyer, Joel R., 65

Ibrahim, Mohab, 64

illness, 12–13, 45, 48, 57–58, 60, 73, 76.
    See also mental health problems; sub-
    stance abuse

Indian Affairs, 22, 24

"Indian problem," 21–22, 66

Indian Territory, 23

Indigenizing/decolonizing efforts, 7, 58–
    62, 71–74, 78

Indigenous epistemologies: and the "be-
    ginning place," 71–72; and connected-
    ness, 6, 30–33, 37–38, 43–44; preced-
    ing Contact, 6, 29–30, 69, 80; and the
    spirit around us, 66–67, 70; synthetic
    nature of, 30–33. See also traditional
    knowledge

Indigenous land rights meeting (2011),
    33–34, 37

individualism, xi, xviii, 21, 37, 54–55

Inuit, 36

Ireland, 40

i tse i (new), 64

Jacobs, Sue-Ellen, 19

James, Jenny, 27

Japan, 64

Johnson, Greg, 34

Johnson-Jennings, Michelle, 80

Judaculla Rock, xix, 41, *42*, 83–84

Junger, Sebastian, 47

Kanane'ski Amayi ehi (Grandmother Wa-
    ter Spider), 17

ka na sa da (not thinking clearly), 74

ka nv wo di (to heal someone), 50

Kilimanjaro, 83

King, Charles, 1–2

Kiowa, 4, 37

Kituwah, North Carolina, xx–xxi, 16–17,
    35, 44–45, 83

Lakota, 63

Lang, Sabine, 19

Las Casas, Bartolomé de, 65

Lefler, Hugh Talmage, 8

Lefler, Jean (Lisa Lefler's mother): and
    Tom Belt, ix–x, xvii–xviii, 12, 64; bo-
    tanical knowledge of, xvi, 15, 34–35,
    76; connection to land, 12, 32, 36, 40,
    43, 64, 74; life of, xv–xvii, 60

Lewis, Courtney, 80

Lewis, Melissa, 80
LGBTQ people, 19–20
Lighthorse, 25
Little Bear, Leroy, 33
Little Big Man (film), 65
Little Tennessee River, 49

Makepeace, Anne, 36–37
Malone, Henry T., 8–9
Mankiller, Wilma, 23
Manning, Maurice, x
Martin-Hill, Dawn, 6, 31
matrilineality: centrality of, to Kituwah,
    17–19, *18*, 24–28; and Mother Earth,
    27, 33; shift away from, 21, 26–27, 66
McCarroll, Meredith, xiv
McLoughlin, William G., 21
Menendez, Pedro, 19
mental health problems: and childhood
    trauma, 56–59; and counseling mod-
    els, 43–44, 46, 55–62; depression, 36,
    44–45, 51, 55, 59; and loss of identity,
    48, 52–53, 77; and mindfulness, 78;
    and stress, 13–14, 56–57, 64, 73. *See
    also* counseling; substance abuse
metaphysics, 30–31, 38, 70
modernization, 53, 83
Mohawk, 20, 38, 68
Momaday, N. Scott, 4–5
Montrose, Louis, 24
moon, 67
Mooney, James, 18
Mother Earth, 27, 33
mountains: connectedness to, xiv–xxi,
    33–34, 43, 82–83; and cosmography,
    xi, 6, 16–17; as "thin places," 40–43,
    83–84. *See also* connectedness; Rooted
    in the Mountains Symposium
Mountains Piled upon Mountains
    (Cory), 7
Mount Juktas, 83

Nan-ye-hi, 25–26
NASA, 33, 66–67

National Institute on Alcohol Abuse and
    Alcoholism, 2
National Public Radio, 37, 64
Native Hawaiians, 34
Native science. *See* traditional knowledge
Native Science Dialogues, 32–33
Native Youth Report, 55
"natural laws," 5, 45–49, 50, 59, 66–67,
    69, 71–72
Navajo, 33, 37, 66, 70
neuroscience, 37–38, 78
Newsome, Albert Ray, 8
New Testament, 71–72, 74
ni gol (i) gv na (not knowing), 73
Nikwasi, 41
nv wo ti (medicine), 50

Obama, Barack, 55
Old Settlers, 23
Otsigiduwagi (people of the Kituwah), 17
Owl, Cliff, 80
Owl, Constance, 80

Palmer, Jane, 20
"Peace of Wild Things, The" (Berry), 1
Peat, F. David, 33
petroglyphs, 41, *42*, 52, 70, 84
Portuguese, 36
"primitive" stereotypes, 2, 30, 32, 49, 54,
    65–66, 79–80
Prucha, Francis Paul, 22
psychology, 6, 14, 20–21, 43–44, 53–54,
    56, 58. *See also* counseling
Pueblo, 67
Puritans, 85

Qualla Boundary, 52
Queen, Mary Jane and Ella, xix–xx

Raleigh, Walter, 24
rattlesnakes, xx
Red Clay, Tennessee, 23
religion: and Cherokee translation
    of New Testament, 71–72, 74;

transformation in, 21, 44; Western, 32, 46, 49, 79. *See also* spirituality

Removal of Native peoples. *See* Cherokee Removal

residential boarding schools, 37, 66

Revolutionary War, 8, 20, 25

Ridge, Major, 69

Riggs, Brett H., 26

Rock, Jim, 33

Rooted in the Mountains Symposium, 16–17, 32–33, 40, 53, 63, 84

Roscoe, Will, 19

Rutherford, Griffith, 25, 49

Sacks, Jonathan, 85

Sagarmatha, 83

Scalice, Daniella, 66

sciences: interconnectedness of, 6–7, 66, 70, 71–72, 75–76; Western under-standings of, 30–33, 37–38, 70, 78

Scolacutta, 25

Scotland, 40

Selhub, Eva, 64

Selu (Corn Mother), 17, 26

Sequoyah, 21

Shenandoah National Park, xiv

Shoemaker, Eugene, 67

Shooting Creek, North Carolina, xx

Skegunsta, Chief, 22

Smith, Herb, xiii

Smithers, Gregory D., 19, 20, 22, 23

social Darwinism, 54

spirituality: and religion, 21, 49, 79; and rootedness, xv, 44, 53, 77; and science, 2, 30–31, 66–70; and women, 26–27. *See also* religion

Spokane Tribe of Indians, 80

sque sta ud'sgwisda (a lot of stuff/sick-ness), 66

Stanford University, 17

stickball, xx, 20

stillness, 43, 81

stomp dance, 48, 51

Strangers and Kin (film), xiii

stress, 13–14, 56–57, 64, 73, 76

substance abuse: alcoholism, xvi, 2, 13–15, 22, 45, 56; and childhood trauma, 58–59; and culturally appropriate treatment, 2, 13–15, 45, 53–55; and Native treatment centers, 55–57, 61–62; pharmaceuticals and, 36. *See also* counseling; mental health problems

suicide, 2, 55–56, 77

tali tsisgwayahi (Two Sparrows Town), 41

ta li tsu da na do gi (two hearts), 19

Taylor, Jill Bolte, 37–38

Tellico Plains, Tennessee, xx

Tennessee Valley Authority, xiii

"thin places," 40–43, 49, 83–84

Thomas, Robert K., 74–75

Thomas, Wesley, 19

thought, power of, 19, 30, 33, 53, 60–61, 76

tikkun olam (acts that make a difference), 85

Timberlake, Henry, 24–25

Time magazine, 37

tohi (health): and balance, 12–13, 36, 48–49, 54, 59–60, 69–70, 76; and cer-emony, 14–15, 60–61, 74; and coming home, xvi–xxi, 45, 50–52; and con-nectedness, 10–11, 36–38, 43, 45, 55, 75, 77–78; and emotions, 73–76, 78; glossed, ix, 5, 10; and "green spaces," 63–64; and Indigenous voices, 2–3, 11–12; and order, 46, 84–85; and prob-lem solving, 51, 73; and spirituality, 66–70; and wholeness, 34–36, 38, 44–45, 59, 74. See also *duyukdv'i/duyu-godvi* (the right path); "natural laws"

Townsend, Dan, *18*

traditional knowledge: centering of, 2–3, 5–7, 80–81, 84; and language, 33, 35, 37, 80; and the medicine in you, 78; scope of, 30; and treatment, 53–54, 57–62. *See also* Indigenous epistemologies

Trafzer, Clifford E., 65

Trail of Tears, xx, 22. *See also* Cherokee Removal

trauma: childhood, 56–59; global amplification of, 85; historical, 14, 20–21, 25, 57, 61, 79–80; and mindfulness, 45, 78

Treaty of New Echota, 69

tribalism, xviii, 43–44, 47, 51, 54, 59–61, 77

Tsanusi, 41

Tsul'kala (Judaculla), 41

Tuscarora Nation, 80

two spirits, 19–20

udohiyu (true reality), 13

ukshaleski (selfishness/it is taken from your anus), 76

Uktena, 41

u la sga ni s di (fool), 74

ulilohi' (things happening as they are "supposed to be"), 63

unalv (anger), 45

une gu tsa da (meanness that came with colonialism), 66

United Keetoowah Band, 16, 23

u tsa ta (intense feelings/pain), 66

Vance, J. D., xiv

vyuga (disease), 45

Wahrhaftig, Albert, 51

Wake Forest University, 33–34

Wampanoag, 36–37

war women, 20, 24

water, 17–18, *18*

Waterrock Knob, 83

Weeks, Guy, 68

Welch, Kevin, 30

well-being. See *tohi* (health)

Werito, Vincent, 70

Western Carolina University, 32–33, 40, 41, 53, 78, 83–84

Western epistemologies: antisynthetic nature of, 30–33, 60, 72, 78; as counterproductive to healing, 35–37, 50, 55–58, 60–62; egocentrism of, 64–67; and fear of unknown, 30, 32, 49, 54, 65–66, 73–74, 79–80. *See also* colonization

We Still Live Here (film), 36–37

Williams, Walter L., 19

Wood, Peter, 19

woodpecker gorget, 17, *18*

Wynne, Melodi, 80

Yellow Bird, Michael, 7, 78, 80

Yonaguska, Chief, 79

Yup'ik, 2